SPEECH AND SONG AT THE MARGINS OF GLOBAL HEALTH

SPEECH AND SONG AT THE MARGINS OF GLOBAL HEALTH

Zulu Tradition, HIV Stigma, and AIDS Activism in South Africa

STEVEN P. BLACK

RUTGERS UNIVERSITY PRESS

New Brunswick, Camden, and Newark, New Jersey, and London

Library of Congress Cataloging-in-Publication Data

Names: Black, Steven P., 1980– author.
Title: Speech and song at the margins of global health : Zulu tradition, HIV stigma,
    and AIDS activism in South Africa / Steven P. Black.
Description: New Brunswick : Rutgers University Press, 2019. | Includes
    bibliographical references.
Identifiers: LCCN 2018057615 | ISBN 9780813597713 (pbk.)
Subjects: LCSH: Sociolinguistics—South Africa. | HIV-positive persons—
    South Africa—Language. | HIV infections—Social aspects—South Africa. |
    Music—Social aspects—South Africa. | Zulu (African people)—
    South Africa—Social conditions. | Stigma (Social psychology)—South Africa. |
    Transmutation (Linguistics) | Choirs (Music)—South Africa.
Classification: LCC P40.45.S6 B53 2019 | DDC 306.4408770968—dc23
LC record available at https://lccn.loc.gov/2018057615

A British Cataloging-in-Publication record for this book is available from the
British Library.

www.rutgersuniversitypress.org

Manufactured in the United States of America

This book is dedicated to the Thembeka choir, members of which opened up their hearts and homes to me. Their courage singing and speaking out about HIV/AIDS has inspired many to action. Their counseling, both informally with community members and formally for AIDS activist organizations, has comforted and informed countless South Africans living with HIV. Any author proceeds will be transferred to the choir and/or donated to South African HIV/AIDS support and activist organizations.

CONTENTS

FIGURES

TRANSCRIPTION CONVENTIONS, ORTHOGRAPHY, AND MORPHEME LABELS

TRANSCRIPTION CONVENTIONS

All transcripts, as representations of actual strips of discourse, cannot fully capture the dynamics of a particular linguistic interchange, let alone the use of gesture, physical space, and body orientation. Rather, transcripts are documents shaped by theory within a particular discipline. As such, thoughtful and theoretically informed choices must be made as to what aspects of an interchange to include in a transcript (Duranti 2006, Ochs 1979). In the excerpts for this paper, the level of descriptive detail in each transcript corresponds with the central analysis being put forward with the transcript. Here are the conventions used in these transcripts (see also Goodwin 1990, Sacks et al. 1974).

((xxx))	Double parentheses encapsulate anything not spoken by the participants, especially a description of gesture, facial expression, body orientation, or the way in which the talk occurred (e.g., singing versus speaking).
:::	Colons show where the sound just prior to the colons has been considerably lengthened.
.	A period indicates a falling intonation.
,	A comma indicates a falling-rising intonation.
?	A question mark indicates a rising intonation.
=	Equal signs indicate when there is no break between the end of one participant's talk and the beginning of another's.
(0.0)	Numbers in single parentheses mark silence in seconds and tenths of seconds.
(xxx)	Words in single parentheses indicates that the transcriber was unsure of the veracity of his/her hearing of the material.

(????)   Question marks in parentheses indicate that something was said, but it is not possible to distinguish the words from a recording.

-           A hyphen indicates a sudden stop in an individual's talk (a glottal stop).

xxx   Underlining indicates emphasis in an individual's talk.

[Right-facing brackets indicate the place where overlap between two or more speakers occurs.

ORTHOGRAPHY

The Zulu language (isiZulu) has a standardized written orthography that is followed here. Orthographic representations and International Phonetic Alphabet (IPA) symbols and descriptions for consonants without equivalents in English are listed in the table.

LETTER	IPA SYMBOL	DESCRIPTION
c	⊙	Dental click
q	ǂ	Palato-alveolar click
x	‖	Alveolar lateral click
hl	ɬ	Voiceless lateral fricative
dl	ɮ	Voiced lateral fricative
h	ʰ	*Aspiration

MORPHEME LABELS

Morpheme labels were produced in consultation with several contemporary and classic isiZulu and Bantu language grammar books (Doke 1930 [1927], Mbeje 2005, Nurse & Philippson 2003, Poulos & Bosch 1997, Poulos & Msimang 1998). The following list includes those labels that are used in the book.

---

* isiZulu distinguishes between voiced, unvoiced, and aspirated consonants. Unless followed by an "l," an "h" indicates aspiration. If followed by an "l," "hl" indicates a voiceless lateral fricative. The absence of an "h" indicates an unvoiced (and unaspirated) consonant.

Nominal class prefixes

SINGULAR	PLURAL
n1 = **u**	n2p = **aba**
n1a = **u**	n2ap = **o**
n3 = **umu**	n4p = **imi**
n5 = **i(li)**	n6p = **ama**
n7 = **isi**	n8p = **izi**
n9 = **in/im**	n10p = **izin/izim**

n11 = **u(lu)** (the plural of n11 is n10p)

n14 = **ubu**

n15 = **uku**

Verbal subject concords

1pl = **si**	1st person plural subject marker
1s = **ngi**	1st person singular subject marker
2pl = **ni**	2nd person plural subject marker
2s = **u**	2nd person singular subject marker
3pl = **ba**	3rd person plural subject marker
3s = **u**	3rd person singular subject marker

SINGULAR	PLURAL
s1 = **u**	s2p = **ba**
s1a = **u**	s2ap = **ba**
s3 = **u**	s4p = **i**
s5 = **li**	s6p = **a**
s7 = **si**	s8p = **zi**
s9 = **i**	s10p = **zi**
s11 = **lu**	

s14 = **bu**

s15 = **ku**

Verbal object concords

o2s = **ku**	2nd person singular object marker
o2p = **ni**	2nd person plural object marker
o# =	Object marker, noun class #

Tense and aspect markers

INDICATIVE MOOD

RmPst = Remote past tense
Pst = Past tense
Pres = present tense
Fut = Future tense
RmFut = Remote future tense

IMPLICATIONS

Indef = Indefinite
Cont = Continuous
Perf = Perfective
Exc = Exclusive

OTHER MOODS

Subj = Subjunctive mood
Part = Participial mood

VERBAL EXTENSIONS

APL = Applicative
CAU = Causative
STA = Stative
PAS = Passive
REF = Reflexive

Rel = Relative affix
Adj = Adjective affix

Demonstratives, possessives, and pronouns

DemAP = demonstrative addressee proximate
DemD = demonstrative distal
DemSP = demonstrative speaker proximate
Pos# = Possessive pronoun, noun class #
P# = Possessive, noun class #
Pro# = Pronoun, noun class #

Other morphemes
  NEG = Negative
  CONJ = Conjunctive formative
  INS = Instrumental formative
  DM = Discourse marker

SPEECH AND SONG AT THE MARGINS
OF GLOBAL HEALTH

1 · INTRODUCTION

It is already dark when we arrive at the funeral. The event is being held at the rural farm of two sisters, Zethu and Amahle, who are members of a unique Zulu gospel choir.[1] The funeral is for their brother. The drive from Durban, a cosmopolitan metropolis and port on the Indian Ocean, to the South African countryside took several hours. So far, what I know of this rural area includes a two-lane road mauled by corporate timber and sugarcane trucks, a tiny town whose main draw is a livestock auction, the dirt wheel-ruts I nervously negotiate in my tiny, two-wheel-drive rental car, and the sound of cows mooing nearby. When I park by a goat shed, five isiZulu-speaking[2] South Africans—members of a gospel choir with whom I have begun to conduct fieldwork—extract themselves from the small car.

On the way to the funeral, a choir member named Fanele had begun to ask me questions about my research. What were my goals? How did I plan to contribute to the activities of the choir? Was I interested in music? Language? HIV/AIDS? She listened carefully to my responses. Then she told me that people living with HIV were tired of researchers who came, asked their questions, and then left. Sometimes, Fanele explained, infected individuals just told researchers what they thought the researchers wanted to hear, took payment, and waited for the researchers to go. If I wanted to know more about what was going on, I would have to stick around.

After we arrive at the farm, I am asked if I want to participate in the evening's events. I nervously reply, "yes," and I am led to the family's roundhouse. The roundhouse is a family ritual center, a large, round, single-room structure with a small Christian altar. Bull horns hang on the wall, and a central post shoots upward to support a conical metal roof. The roundhouse is a space to commune with one's ancestors during family events, such as deaths, births, and birthdays. It had once been the one-room home of the family before a larger, rectangular house with bedrooms, a living room, and a kitchen had been built. Days before the funeral, the body and soul of the deceased had been carefully led by a spiritual leader, Baba Shangane, to the roundhouse from a township near Durban.

From outside, I can hear a number of people singing Zulu hymns. I have no idea what to expect. I have never been to a Zulu funeral before. I take a deep breath and walk into the room. It is like jumping into cold water. I feel out of place. Fifty pairs of eyes look up at me.

The father of the deceased, who I would later learn to call Baba (father), quickly pulls up a plastic chair and kindly asks me to sit next to him. The hymns continue. Baba is a black South African man who lived through both the official beginning of apartheid in 1948 and its legislative dismantling in 1994. He labored in the manufacturing industry and worked with his brothers to maintain the family farm where I now sit. He also saved up to buy and maintain a four-room, government-built, cinder-block home in a formerly black township near Durban, where Amahle and Zethu now live with their sister, their nephew, and Zethu's son. In the early 2000s, at a time when some parents disowned children who disclosed their HIV-positive status, Baba had responded with compassion and love upon hearing the news that two of his daughters were HIV positive. Though I did not learn this until later on, his son, whom he is burying at this funeral, died as a result of HIV infection.

In the familial roundhouse, knee-to-knee and shoulder-to-shoulder with Baba, I glance around the room. I notice that all the men who are present sit on chairs or benches, whereas the women sit on mats on the floor. These observations are interrupted by a question:

"Why are you not singing?" Baba asks in English. "Are you not Christian?"

"I don't know these songs in Zulu," I respond, answering the first question and evading the next. My answer seems to satisfy him. With each song, funeral-goers seamlessly weave their voices together in four-part harmony. When one hymn ends, someone in the group takes the initiative and begins the next song. The effect is almost hypnotic. Minutes and hours disappear over a temporal horizon, replaced by the rhythmic cycles of song into which participants immerse themselves. After a number of songs have begun and ended, Amahle asks me if I would like to go and sleep. She leads me to her father's bed. She explains that neither he nor the others would sleep that night, but that it would be inappropriate for me to be present for some of the night's events. So, I sleep.

In the morning after I awaken, I sit quietly in a small living room watching Amahle, Zethu, and other women prepare breakfast. Two couches create a border around a cowhide rug that lies over a polished concrete floor. In the corner, a small black-and-white TV is attached to what appears to be a car battery. There is no electricity in the house, no toilet, and no municipal water, but a gas stove (fueled by paraffin) and a large water tank ensure that the kitchen is a comfortable space in which to cook. I look out a window and see some men on the edge of a cornfield, taking turns using a pickax and shovel to dig a grave.

Soon, one man comes to find me in the house. He invites me to come with him, instructing me, "No Steve—you mustn't sit with the women here. Come and sit with the men outside." I go with him. I try to interact with the other men, even though at this early point in my fieldwork I am not a fluent isiZulu speaker. However, many of the men speak English. At one point, someone sits down with me and asks where I am from.

"Oh, you're American," he muses. "Where is your camera? Don't you have a camera?"

"No," I reply. "Well, I do have a camera, but I wasn't sure about using it. I just wasn't sure if it was appropriate or not, and I was even afraid to ask because I thought it would be disrespectful."

He zeroes in on the word "disrespectful," quickly responding, "Ah, that's good. That shows that you already know something about Zulu culture."

Later, as I stand talking with that man and a few older men, he exclaims, "You see, Steve is here with his heart. He didn't come with his video camera to shoot pictures and then take them back to America. He came here with his heart to experience our culture." This statement about coming first and foremost as a person to experience and understand the lives of others would stay with me throughout my research.

The daytime funeral service is held inside a large, white vinyl tent pitched next to the house. Amid the ethos of "living positively" maintained by the Thembeka choir, the funeral is a reminder of the constant stream of tragedies in a nation where as much as 20 percent of the population may be infected with HIV. Rows of white plastic chairs face an open casket, in front of which a number of pastors and religious leaders from various groups take turns sermonizing. At this funeral, unlike many American funerals, any religious leader who wishes to speak is free to do so. From the rear of the tent, I watch and listen as the coffin is shut and Amahle, sister of the deceased, calls out in lament.

After he died, Amahle and Zethu found a shoebox full of unopened anti-retroviral medication (ARV) under their brother's bed. He had been going to collect the medication but not taking it. Presumably the act of going to the clinic was meant to satisfy his activist sisters that he was receiving treatment. The tragedy of his passing was compounded by the knowledge that the death might have been prevented. In one family, in one home, three siblings were living with HIV. Why did one sibling reject medical treatment while the other two thrived?

OVERVIEW

I traveled to Durban, South Africa, in early February 2008, to stay for a period of nine months, conducting ethnographic fieldwork on language, music, culture, and HIV/AIDS. Upon arrival, I hoped to focus my research on a choir consisting of people living with HIV. The choir, called the Thembeka choir, was part support group, part activist organization, and part performance troupe. The choir had been on tour five times to the United States and once to England, the trips paid for by an international Christian aid group and donations. The choir could be labeled a biosocial group—that is, a group in which membership is in part dependent on a shared biomedically defined characteristic (in this case, diagnosis with HIV infection) (Rabinow 1992). Combining this concept of the biosocial group with linguistic anthropology's notion of the speech community, in this book I describe the choir as a bio-speech community to help model how the choir community intersected with other groups (e.g., biomedical research organizations, activist groups, Christian aid groups) that shared biomedical orientations toward HIV/AIDS (see Bucholtz 1999; Eckert and McConnell-Ginet 1998 for critiques of the speech community concept; more to come on this). When I began fieldwork, I was interested in the choir because it was an instance of an intervention that seems to be succeeding amid the many disappointments of the South African epidemic. I was hoping to complete what Joel Robbins (2013) later theorized as "an anthropology of the good"; though as fieldwork progressed

I learned that the choir's situation was more ambivalent and complex than I had initially imagined. I was also interested in the choir because this success-ful intervention involved music. I arrived in Durban with twenty-three years of musical training, including fifteen years of work as a jazz saxophone player and an undergraduate degree in ethnomusicology. Like other researchers before me (e.g., Barz 2006; McNeill 2011), I planned to use music as an eth-nographic research tool in settings around HIV/AIDS. Prior to my arrival, I had also studied anthropology (earning a B.A. and an M.A. in the field), spe-cializing in the subfields of linguistic and medical anthropology. One of my research goals was to understand how members of the Thembeka choir used language and music to construct support and engage in HIV activism amid the intense stigma that characterized the South African AIDS epidemic. Nine months of fieldwork also resulted in learning about research participants' translinguistic practices—that is, how they incorporated multiple linguistic codes into a hybrid communicative toolkit (García 2009; Reynolds and Ore-llana 2015)—to *transpose* biomedical models of HIV across the borders of multiple communities at the margins of global health (more to come on this).

This book synthesizes theoretical lenses from linguistic, medical, and psychological anthropology to advance a new perspective on the activities, roles, and positioning of marginalized aid recipients in global health. This per-spective emerged out of my encounters with members of the Thembeka choir. When I traveled to Durban, South Africa, in 2008 to study communi-cation, culture, and HIV/AIDS stigma, I expected to hear stories of death, despair, exclusion, and suffering; such stories were indeed prominent. How-ever, the choir promoted a different outlook—one rooted in play and cre-ativity. At choir rehearsals and social gatherings, group members sang songs together about HIV and Christian faith. They also told stories and joked with one another about HIV. Vocal play was interconnected with play (in the nom-inal sense of the word) in the choir's structural positioning at the borders of both global health and Durban-area communities. Located at the margins of several networks, the Thembeka choir was paradoxically at the center of mul-tiple overlapping speech communities associated with global health in Dur-ban. While members of these communities (including the choir community) came from numerous distinct ethnic, racial, class, educational, and national backgrounds, one thing that provided a place of contact and overlap was a set of biomedical perspectives toward HIV/AIDS. Linking anthropological schol-arship on biosociality and biopower with research on speech communities and biocommunicability, I coin the term "bio-speech communities" to emphasize research participants' shared orientations toward powerful biomedical perspectives on HIV/AIDS.

Through performance in speech and song, specifically by *transposing* AIDS across social and cultural contexts, choir members worked to create the social and economic space not only to exist but also to thrive at the margins of global health at a time when many other infected individuals were depressed or dying. Here, I adapt the term "transposition" from musical terminology (cf. Jakobson 1959: 238; Silverstein 2003). I use the term as a way to link research in medical and psychological anthropology on explanatory models/medical pluralism and the "translation" of scientific objects with scholarship in linguistic anthropology on code-switching/translanguaging. Generally, to transpose means to move an entity from one context or setting to another. In music, specifically, to transpose means to shift a song from one harmonic center (or key) to another. While each transposed performance includes the same melody and harmony, the shift in harmonic center may give the same song a different feel (e.g., as one moves from the bass tones of one harmonic center to the treble tones of another, or vice versa). In jazz music, performers sometimes improvise or plan such transpositions in the midst of a song as a way to shift the feel of the performance. Analogously, while the core meaning of biomedical terminology remained the same when Thembeka choir members used biomedical terminology in distinct linguistic (English and isiZulu) and community contexts (in choir rehearsals, at a research clinic, in encounters with other support group members), a shift in the indexical and semantic significance of words sometimes occurred.

While this book analyzes the language of HIV support and activism in South Africa, the lessons learned from the analysis may be applicable to many global health contexts, and to examinations of marginality and international aid more broadly. Drawing from research on globalization and science–technology–society studies, anthropologists emphasize that global health comprises complex networks of circulating discourses, money, technologies, medicine, people, and pathogens (Biehl and Petryna 2013; Brada 2017; Fassin 2012; Nguyen 2010). Within and among networks, the circulation of these resources, discourses, people, and pathogens is uneven. The linguistic anthropological theorizations of play and performance that are utilized in this book place the actions of marginalized persons at the center of the analysis, demonstrating how such persons engage with, and in some cases transform, the overlapping community-wide, national, and transnational institutional and societal structures that have marginalized them.

This ethnography is based on fieldwork conducted in Durban, South Africa. With over two million inhabitants in the greater metropolitan area, Durban is the largest city in the province of KwaZulu-Natal (figure 1.1). The city is home to the second-busiest port in Africa (after Port Said, Egypt) and is the epicenter of the South African AIDS epidemic. In 2008, by some estimates, as much as 35 percent of adult residents of reproductive age in the province were HIV positive, and 10.6 percent of South Africans were HIV positive (Shisana et al. 2009). In other words, Durban is deeply enmeshed in patterns of inter- and intranational circulation associated with global capitalism, global health, and the AIDS pandemic. About the pandemic, a Joint United Nations Programme on HIV/AIDS (UNAIDS) report indicates that in the mid-2000s AIDS was the worldwide leading cause of death among persons aged 15–19 and remained the leading cause of death in Africa through 2010 (cited in Bulled 2015: 20). The International AIDS Conference has been held twice in Durban, first in 2000 and then in 2016. By 2012, the national estimate for HIV prevalence had gone up to 12.2 percent, and KwaZulu-Natal remained the state with the most infections (Shisana et al. 2014). These statistics and the conference's location are an indication that Durban has been not only an epicenter of the pandemic but also a central location for global health researchers, scholars, doctors, and media professionals interested in HIV/AIDS.

As in other global health contexts, Durban global health in 2008 included a dizzying array of interests, institutions, and actors, including the South African National Department of Health, government-run and private hospitals, South African nonprofit organizations (including activist organizations such as LoveLife and the Treatment Action Campaign [TAC]), international nonprofit organizations, the World Health Organization (WHO), UNAIDS, The Bill and Melinda Gates Foundation, and the U.S. President's Emergency Plan for AIDS Relief (PEPFAR). For people living with HIV, many of these groups provided potential access to money, medication, and treatment. Many members of the Thembeka choir were active in multiple HIV/AIDS organizations focused on prevention, treatment, and activism, and the choir itself was an outgrowth of these organizations and efforts. These governmental and nongovernmental institutions also provided communicative and ideological links to global health that were significant as an alternative to the HIV stigma that many infected individuals experienced in their home and work life.

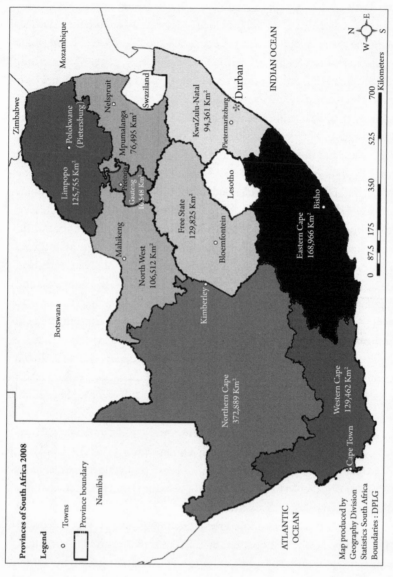

FIGURE 1.1. Provinces of South Africa, modified by Steven P. Black, original from Statistics South Africa 2008. All images by Steven P. Black unless otherwise noted.

Researcher Positionality

This research project presented a number of challenges and opportunities with respect to my positioning among research participants, public health researchers, and scholars. First, in conducting this research I have struggled with the question of research participant anonymity with regard to the publications and artistic products of other researchers. In my research, I use pseudonyms to refer to people and organizations. This was both stipulated in institutional review board (IRB) documents and agreed upon in consultation with choir members. At the outset of my fieldwork in 2008, it seemed to me that anonymity needed to be maintained amid the intense stigmatization of HIV in South Africa. My decision to use pseudonyms contrasts with the American documentary filmmakers and with another scholar who conducted research with the choir prior to my arrival. These scholars use choir members' real names in publications. This puts me in the awkward position of being required not to cite their work, because to do so would be to effectively reveal group members' identities. I am uncertain what the actual motivation was for their use of group members' real names, but I do know that on multiple occasions several research participants insisted to me that they were okay with their real names appearing in print. Still, when I had an in-depth discussion about pseudonyms with choir members in 2013, the outcome of our conversation was that anonymity should be maintained (this encounter is discussed in chapter 6). The question of how and when to disclose, if at all, is a core moral/ethical dilemma posed by the overlapping exigencies of global health ideologies and Zulu tradition theorized in this book. Here, I have chosen to prioritize the ethics of my consent process (maintaining anonymity) over the ethics of scholarship (appropriate citation).

Also evident in this book are concerns regarding the power dynamic between researcher and research participant. For many years, scholars in feminist studies and black studies have "exposed the way that being studied by 'white men' (to use a shorthand for a complex and historically constituted subject-position) turns into being spoken for by them" (Abu-Lughod 1991: 142–143). Indeed, the question of how to go about being a white, American, middle-class man studying black, marginalized, South Africans (predominantly women), always significant, was foregrounded in my experiences at the funeral recounted in the prologue of this book. At the funeral, it became clear that I was not the first researcher—and in particular not the first American researcher—to visit Amahle's extended family at their rural farm. The question, "You're American—where's your camera?" hinted at something I later learned more about. A group of American film students had traveled to South Africa and filmed a documentary about the choir that included a visit to Amahle and Zethu's family farm. Additionally, my conversation with Fanele, in which she stated that people living with HIV were tired of researchers, indicated that she and others had already been in contact with a number of doctors and scholars from South Africa and abroad. In fact, alongside an Ivy League American doctor named Laura, Fanele co-led an innovative testing and treatment organization. Through such points of contact, marginalized South Africans living with HIV worked to access the uneven global circulation of money, medicine, and knowledge that shaped the AIDS pandemic. And through this contact, participants had formed ideas about researchers like me.

My positioning as an American with respect to that of stigmatized research participants was also a source of opportunities for communication and exchange. Thembeka choir members and other research participants often thought of Americans as people less likely to stigmatize HIV. In addition, being a foreigner meant that I was less likely to inadvertently disclose research participants' HIV status through nonresearch social contact with home communities because I was not initially a part of those communities. Also, when I analyze the Thembeka choir as a centrally positioned bio-speech community amid overlapping, transnationally situated groups associated with global health, I consider myself a part of these groups. Though I was indeed an outsider in group members' township communities and in South African academic circles, as an American researcher I followed transnational patterns of movement associated with global health. To position myself as Other with respect to the choir would mean to ignore the complexities of global circulation that indirectly linked me to the group (cf. Jacobs-Huey 2002; Narayan 1993).

This book is focused substantially on research participants' engagements with multiple groups and institutions associated with global health. My own experiences with those communities were mixed. For instance, early in 2008 I contacted Durban Hospital (the Thembeka choir had been affiliated with the hospital's clinic) to ask them about conducting fieldwork with the choir and with the hospital. The hospital asked me to submit study documents to their newly established IRB. After I submitted the study documents, I was invited to a meeting with IRB members. At the meeting, I received no substantial critiques of the methods or ethics of the study. Instead, I was informed that people who were allowed to conduct research at the hospital were those who "stuck around for a while" (similar to what Fanele had told me). However, unlike with the choir, the hospital denied me access. Since my National Science Foundation funding was limited to nine months, I did not see conducting research with the hospital as a feasible option.

I was also worried by another comment made by one of the IRB members. One doctor told me that the choir would be unable to understand my research project well enough to make their own decision about allowing access and consenting to the research. She said that I should take the hospital's rejection as a rejection of conducting fieldwork with the choir as well, even though the choir was technically no longer affiliated with the hospital. This comment struck me as indicating a patronizing attitude toward the choir (months later, when I confided in Zethu with this story, she was shocked that the hospital staff thought they could speak for the choir). In general, my encounters with South African public health researchers were not easy. I struggled to reconcile their top-down approach to biomedical research with my anthropological commitment to understanding health and illness from the bottom up—that is, starting from the concerns and perspectives of infected individuals, rather than imposing the priorities of biomedicine.

I decided to ignore the IRB's advice, and soon after I met with choir leaders Thulani and Philani at a café in downtown Durban. As we sat sipping our lattes in a faux-leather booth at the busy coffee shop, the choir leaders (both men) told me that they had worked with many researchers before (like Fanele had said), appeared in documentaries, and gone on tour five times to the United States and once to England, at no cost to themselves, in order to increase AIDS awareness and raise money, yet they were still poor. They explained that they knew I was a student and that I therefore did not have much money, but that they expected contributions—not necessarily monetary—in exchange for their participation. I interpreted their discussion out loud: "You do not want to be taken advantage of?" Yes, they replied. This exchange pointed to some of the complexities that I would later explore in terms of choir members' contacts with other researchers and the structural inequities of global aid, activism, and research.

TOWARD A THEORIZATION OF TRANSPOSITION AND BIO-SPEECH COMMUNITIES

In the remaining chapters of this book, I contribute to a growing body of literature at the intersection of linguistic and medical anthropology (Briggs and Faudree 2016) with a discussion of the role of linguistic and musical performance in the constitution of support and activism in global health amid stigma. This places the book at the margins of multiple subdisciplinary boundaries, focusing on the bridging of distinct but overlapping theorizations of culture, language, performance, and social life. This body of work has roots that are at least thirty years old. In early research on the subject, Joel Kuipers (1989) identifies three ways of understanding "medical discourse." One viewpoint, often employed by doctors but also shared by some medical anthropologists, is the commonsense notion that language can be a tool for facilitating rapport (e.g., bedside manner, a method for translating between biomedical discourse [of doctors] and the [cultural] outlook of a patient) and for precise reference (reference to entities such as viruses and bodies, or to the inner states and thoughts of a speaker). Although it is perhaps productive in the training of biomedical doctors, Kuipers suggests that this viewpoint is out of touch with rigorous analysis of how language and discourse function and how meaning-making actually occurs. A second viewpoint, derived from poststructuralist philosophy and from the work of Michel Foucault in particular, emphasizes that biomedical discourse wields a powerful force (biopower) that defines the scope of possibilities for talking about and perceiving the living body, thereby shaping individual subjectivities (more to come on biopower). Though useful, this viewpoint often eschews discussion of actual language use in favor of a more broadly defined concept of discourse that consists of all the dominant ways of speaking about medicine, health, and illness. A third viewpoint—an application of microanalytic techniques of conversation analysis—examines the emergent moment-to-moment progression of medical encounters and the ways that language is used to produce social actions in biomedicine. While also useful, this viewpoint often (but not always—see Stivers 2007 for a counterexample) focuses narrowly on moments of language use to the exclusion of large-scale sociohistorical patterns. Twenty years later, James Wilce's (2009b) assessment of the field is similar to Kuipers's. However, Wilce also identifies key terms that have helped scholars to synthesize viewpoints two and three and move

beyond them. Significantly, these key terms include "genre," "global circulation," and "intertextuality."

This book contributes the concepts of bio-speech communities and transposition to this toolkit to further new perspectives at the intersection of
linguistic and medical anthropology (see also Briggs and Mantini-Briggs
2016; Carr 2010; Guzmán 2014; Harvey 2013; Parkin 2013; Pritzker 2014).
Here, I draw from a set of theoretical concepts in three core areas where there
is overlap between linguistic and medical anthropology. The first is reflexivity: I link research on reflexive language with research on reflexivity in
thought, focusing especially on the dynamics of embodied reflexivity in vocal
performance in speech and song. The second is global circulation: I connect
scholarship on the global circulation of discourses/language with scholarship on global circulation (of money, people, medicine, and other resources)
in public/global health contexts. The third is community: I juxtapose literature
on the constitution of sociality in biomedical contexts (biosociality) with
literature on the role of speech and language in the constitution of communities. These three key concepts—reflexivity, circulation, and community—
provide the foundation for the exploration of the concepts of bio-speech
community and transposition. Transposition theorizes how, at the margins of
global health and amid threats of stigmatization, a bio-speech community
consisting of Thembeka choir members and other South African patient-
activists relied on biomedical terminology and a stable biomedical model of
HIV/AIDS as they moved across the margins of the distinct but overlapping
groups associated with global health. Here, I provide a brief overview of the
three key concepts and introduce the ideas of bio-speech communities and
transposition that are further developed throughout the book.

Embodied Reflexivity in Performance

All medical discourse is performance in the sense that all language use is a
performance. However, in many healing traditions, semiotic resources are
organized into patterns of rhythm, melody, harmony, and entrainment that
correspond with more narrowly defined performance genres, sometimes
defined with the umbrella concept of ethnopoetics (Koen et al. 2008; Webster and Kroskrity 2013). It is this more restricted definition of performance
that I utilize in this book. Whether in speech or song, the semiotic grounding for vocal performance is both profoundly social and at the same time
deeply personal (Feld et al. 2004; Turino 1999). The embodied rhythmic

entrainment of performers producing sound together, and in the process synchronizing their experience of time with each other and with audiences, provides a strong intersubjective grounding for social support, healing, and care (Schutz 1964).

Reflexivity and subjunctivity—the imaginative consideration of the way things might be—are defining features of performance (Turner 1987). Performers reflexively attend to their own communicative actions as a key part of the interpretation of meaning, alongside concurrent attention and evaluation by audiences (Bauman 1975; Berger and Del Negro 2002). Increased attention to the poetics of language and music is correlated with increased semantic ambiguity, as persons search for meaning in the patterning of linguistic choices and repetitions (Feld and Fox 1994; Jakobson 1960). In health contexts, the linguistic reflexivity of performance is often linked to moral/ethical reflection upon health, illness, and caregiving. Healing performances include illness narratives (stories about illness), laments about illness, and the musical/vocal patterning of caregiving. Though not often described as performance by medical anthropologists, analyses of illness narratives have figured prominently in anthropological discussions of health (e.g., Brenneis 1988; Capps and Ochs 1995; Kleinman 1988; Mattingly and Garro 2000). Lament is also common in healing performance traditions, where thinking, feeling, and sociability coalesce (Briggs 1993; Wilce 2009a, 2017). Many healing traditions, including those that incorporate lament, also employ vocal/musical performance as part of the therapeutic process (Desjarlais 1992; Koen 2005). This may be because the aesthetic and reflexive contours of specific healing genres help ill individuals to embody the psychological flexibility to disengage, reflect upon their options, and select the best option to move beyond negative understandings of illness (Hinton and Kirmayer 2017).

From a phenomenological standpoint, the communicative activities of healing are simultaneously social action and embodied experience (Ochs 2012). Such activities often fall somewhere in the middle of a continuum of reflexivity. On that continuum, everyday habitual (communicative) acts fall toward one end, and conscious (often linguistically articulated) reflection on what one has done or will do falls toward the other end. Vocal performance in speech and song is often significant in the production of intermediate, not fully coherent experiences of embodied reflection (Throop 2003: 235). In the chapters that follow, I discuss the ways that Thembeka choir members joked about HIV, told stories about HIV, and sang songs about HIV. I examine how the embodied reflexivity of these performances (on stage and in everyday life) contributed to the maintenance of a support group as choir members navigated the overlapping communities associated with global health. I also analyze how biomedical terminology was incorporated into these types of performance, how such performances impacted global health, and how the embodied enactment of these performances played a role in the constitution of a bio-speech community.

Uneven Global Circulation and Biocommunicability

The Thembeka choir's global positioning provides for linkages between the preceding theorization of the embodied reflexivity of performance with scholarship on the uneven transnational circulation of people, goods, and services associated with global health. Studies of globalization assert that transnational circulation across national and regional borders is uneven, shaped by the contours of globalized inequality and the conflicts or friction that arises (Ong and Collier 2008). Dichotomized borders of center versus periphery, urban versus rural, and cosmopolitan versus local belie a complex interpenetration of the global in the local (and vice versa). In now-classic research, Arjun Appadurai (1996) theorizes uneven, interrelated, multiple global circulations with the metaphor of landscapes, examining ethnoscapes (people), mediascapes (media), technoscapes (technology), financescapes (money), and ideoscapes (ideas) (33). Note that language, especially in terms of the grammatical structures that shape circulation of language across discursive and linguistic borders, is implicit in a number of these scapes but is largely unanalyzed by Appadurai. Research on medical humanitarianism and global health in southern Africa repurposes this metaphor of contoured landscapes, using the term "medicoscapes" to discuss how medicine, caregiving, and medical discourses circulate and how that circulation impacts the lives of southern African patients and health workers (Hörbst and Gerrits 2016). Other scholarship describes biomedical circulation in terms of global "assemblages" (Nguyen 2008). In such anthropological models of globalization and health, medicine, money, medical discourses, doctors, global health professionals, researchers, and activists circulate unevenly within and across national borders in conjunction with and in response to the uneven circulation associated with global capitalism.

Developed at the intersection of linguistic and medical anthropology, the concept of biocommunicability theorizes the role of language in this uneven circulation across borders associated with public health and global health. Not only patients but also medical practitioners draw from cultural models (including dominant biomedical models) to understand illness and engage in healing. The term "biocommunicable models" refers to cultural models about health communication, especially models about how health discourse (e.g., medical terms, phrases, ways of speaking about illness, epidemiological data) could or should circulate (Briggs 2011). In reality, health discourse circulates among patients, doctors, epidemiologists, and others in ways that are complex and nonlinear. However, some biocommunicable models simplify or obscure this complexity (Briggs and Hallin 2016: 7).

One of the most consequential biocommunicable models associated with global health is a top-down model of authoritative biomedical discourse. In this model, patients' objectified, biomedicalized bodies are a source of raw data for medical studies and epidemiological reports. Expert doctors, epidemiologists, and researchers produce reports that are then transmitted back to patients (top down) in the form of guidelines, recommendations, and treatment regimens. Such a model erases patient-activist agency and input. For instance, Charles Briggs and Clara Mantini-Briggs (2016) describe a rabies epidemic among indigenous Venezuelan children that was not properly diagnosed due to doctors' negligence in listening to or probing aspects of parent narratives about their children's illness that fell outside of standardized medical routines. In that case, reliance on a top-down biocommunicable model changed the course of the epidemic by preventing doctors from collecting relevant epidemiological information such that public health officials did not pursue an intervention of vaccination. In this book, I will discuss how a similar top-down biocommunicable model marginalized patient-activists from global health groups, limiting patient-activists' ability to collaborate with global health professionals.

Bio-Speech Communities

The ubiquity of authoritative biomedical models in contemporary global health and public discourses is just one indication of the power of biomedicine in shaping persons' perspectives and actions in contemporary contexts (Foucault 1965 [1961]). One aspect of this power is the distinct configuration of roles and relationships oriented around shared biomarkers or biological experiences—what has been termed biosociality (Rabinow 1992). For instance, an HIV support group (or choir) could be considered a biosocial group because it is a group created and maintained in dialogue with biomedical knowledge of the human immunodeficiency virus, including the ability of doctors to detect the virus in individuals. Indeed, medical anthropologists discuss biosociality with respect to medical conditions such as diabetes and HIV, examining how individuals reconfigure notions of self and social group in response to their diagnoses (Guell 2011; Marsland 2012). While linguistic practices are central to the constitution and maintenance of such groups, language is undertheorized in research on biosociality (but see Friedner 2010). This book contributes to such scholarship with the development of the bio-speech communities concept.

The notion of bio-speech communities theorizes the role of language and communication in biosociality by synthesizing research on biosociality and biocommunicability with scholarship on speech communities (see Morgan 2004 for a history of the speech community concept). John Gumperz's (1972) ethnography of speaking approach is a classic and useful starting point for my own discussion of speech community. While scholars have critiqued Gumperz's assumptions of relative homogeneity and consensus among group members (among other criticisms) (e.g., Bucholtz 1999), these assumptions are quite effective in modeling the strong centralizing force of biopower and biosociality—especially amid threats of stigmatization—on group formation. Gumperz defines a speech community by three attributes: (1) regular and frequent interaction, (2) a shared verbal repertoire, and (3) shared social norms of language use (later reinterpreted by some as shared language ideologies). More recent work has interrogated each of these three attributes and, in some cases, offered alternative terms, such as "speech network" and "community of practice" that better model the heterogeneity, complexity, and internal distinctions of groups of people that speak to one another (e.g., Bucholtz 1999; Milroy 2002). In some cases, interaction may be mediated— for instance, in shared linguistic engagement with media (Spitulnik 1996); in some instances, community members may not share a language in common but instead orient toward shared narratives of place and community, described as a "narrated community" (Falconi 2013); and some communities may hold divergent ideologies about language use (Morgan 2001). In communities oriented around heritage languages or endangered languages, on the other hand, metalinguistic attitudes or ideologies may be what holds groups together when individuals have little actual mastery of a heritage/ endangered language, described as a "metalinguistic community" (Avineri 2017, Avineri and Kroskrity 2014). Meanwhile, recent scholarship emphasizes the processual nature of group formation and the transience and instability of communities in the midst of the types of global circulation mentioned earlier (Blommaert 2013; Lønsmann et al. 2017). The sum of this contemporary scholarship is a view of Gumperz's three attributes as a constellation of features that are important for the maintenance of heterogeneous communities with porous boundaries, where one or more of these features may be altered or contested in any particular group of people.

While many contemporary speech activities may not include all three of these features of the speech community concept, the Thembeka choir actually aligned very closely with this classic conceptualization. The analysis presented in this book suggests that biopower, biosociality, and biocommunicability— in short, the unique authority of biomedical discourses—constituted the key reason for this group's alignment with the speech community concept. Group members met frequently, and many saw one another outside of choir contexts in their roles as friends, neighbors, HIV counselors, and global health activists. They had a shared verbal repertoire that was distinguished from others' repertoires, especially in the ways that they narrated, joked about, and sang about HIV, as well as how they transposed HIV across languages and contexts. Finally, choir members maintained (to a certain extent) shared language ideologies, especially in the ways that they valued, embodied, and enacted HIV disclosure, and the ways that they emphasized biomedical terminology and biomedical conceptualizations of HIV. At the same time, there were limits to this consensus—limits that are also explored and discussed in the book.

In other words, this speech community was created and maintained primarily through patterns of communication that were biosocial in nature. In conjunction with the almost unparalleled power and authority of biomedical discourse in many contemporary contexts, I suggest that it is useful to think of the Thembeka choir—and other similar groups—as a bio-speech community. With the idea of bio-speech communities developed in this book, I argue both that theorizations of biosociality do not sufficiently examine the role of language use or language ideologies in constituting biosocial groups, and that the speech community concept must be broadened to recognize the significance of biopower in processes of group formation and maintenance in biomedical contexts. Health inequities and communicative inequities are co-constitutive (Briggs and Mantini-Briggs 2016). Particular communities of people who speak nondominant languages, who employ nonstandard communicative conventions, and who have limited access to authority, may be ignored, silenced, or otherwise left out of the circulation of health discourses and resources. Communicative exclusion may shape the course of an epidemic by changing diagnoses and decisions about how available medicine and treatment are distributed. In this book, I detail how choir members' transposition of biomedical terminology and models across social activities and communities challenged such marginalization. This book examines the formation and maintenance of a bio-speech community at the borders of (1) global health groups, from which they were partially excluded; and (2) other South African communities, from which they were also partially excluded due to stigma. The Thembeka choir's formation at the margins of multiple organizations and institutions meant that the group was positioned at the center of the space where these global health groups overlapped.

Transposition as a Special Case of Translanguaging

In this book, I take the unusual step of using the term "transposition" rather than "code-mixing," "code-switching," or "borrowing." In addition to the inspiration provided by uses of the term in music, I adapt "transposition" from work by Roman Jakobson (1959) on poetics/ verbal art and translation. There, Jakobson suggests that poetry can never truly be translated; rather, "only creative transposition is possible: either intralingual transposition— from one poetic shape into another, or interlingual transposition—from one language into another, or finally intersemiotic transposition—from one system of signs into another, e.g. from verbal art into music, dance, cinema, or painting" (238). Following Jakobson's lead, I use transposition to describe how choir members and other patient-activists retained a stable conceptualization of HIV/AIDS as they moved through multiple communities and across multiple languages (English and isiZulu).

Transposition was a key communicative practice that helped define the choir bio-speech community. Here, I model transposition as both a special case of "translanguaging" (García 2009) and as one possible configuration of medical pluralism (Baer 2011). Whereas conversational codeswitching refers to a speaker's use of two or more language varieties within a speech event or exchange (Woolard 2004: 73–74), translanguaging reconceptualizes code-switching to foreground speakers' integration of multiple codes into a hybrid toolkit that responds to and plays with existing ideological stances toward language varieties (Reynolds and Orellana 2015: 318–319). The concept of transposition combines linguistic anthropology's close analysis of communicative practices in translanguaging with medical anthropology's focus on the cultural models that shape persons' understandings of illness.

In this book, transposition describes how English terminology, ideologically laminated onto biomedical conceptualizations of HIV/AIDS, was utilized by research participants across communities and across language varieties. This builds on previous scholarship about how scientific objects are "translated" across both cultural and linguistic boundaries (e.g., Langwick 2007; Pigg 1997, 2001). In their discussions of HIV/AIDS, whether in English, isiZulu, or some mixture of the two, Thembeka choir members usually did not translate biomedical terminology. Rather, they used English to refer to HIV/AIDS and related concepts across linguistic contexts and communities. In health-seeking behaviors more generally, each research participant idiosyncratically drew from three explanatory models of illness—biomedicine, Christian faith healing, and southern African traditional medicine—in ways that have been described with concepts such as explanatory frameworks and medical pluralism (see Baer 2011; Buchbinder 2011, Garro 2000, Penkala-Gawecka and Rajtar 2016, Scourgie 2008). However, in their actions and discussions related to HIV specifically, all group members maintained an ideological commitment to biomedical explanations and treatment. Despite this commitment, the shift of communicative context altered the meaning of HIV terminology in subtle ways. For instance, in rehearsals, medical terms indexed an AIDS activist stance (in opposition to stigmatizing terms), while in a research meeting with global health professionals the same terms were taken for granted as representative of empirical truth. The concept of transposition connects linguistic anthropology's work on code-switching and translanguaging to medical anthropology and biomedical discussions of medical pluralism. It models the (sometimes improvisatory) linguistic and health-seeking actions undertaken amidst larger-scale patterns of medical pluralism. Choir members used English medical terminology in English and in isiZulu as they moved from discussions about HIV with global health professionals to researchers, from neighbors and family members to Christian aid workers.

While choir members did not usually translate biomedical terms related to HIV/AIDS, linguistic anthropological scholarship on translation nonetheless provides guidance on how to analyze their transposition of biomedical terminology. Such scholarship emphasizes that translation is not a simple process of finding the words in one language that correspond to the referential content in another. Rather, meanings may subtly or dramatically shift as speakers respond to the exigencies of the social, communicative, and semiotic contexts of translation (e.g., Hanks 2010; Pritzker 2014; Schieffelin 2007). Silverstein (2003) theorizes this sort of shift in meaning using the term "semiotic transduction," a term that has become popular in recent years. Transposition could be described as a specific kind of semiotic transduction involving translanguaging accompanied by an effort to retain a coherent cultural model across linguistic contexts.[3] Indeed, Thembeka choir members worked to maintain a core set of biomedical meanings associated with HIV across linguistic contexts. However, subtle shifts akin to those of translation nonetheless occurred as biomedical terminology was adapted to each distinct social and communicative context.

The Thembeka choir and other patient-activists living with HIV maintained a strong ideological connection between English biomedical terminology, the rejection of HIV stigma, and an embrace of global health. While generalized English code-mixing/borrowing in choir members' isiZulu conversations was not necessarily an indication of outlook or understanding, choir members' specific use of English biomedical terminology involved the transfer of a coherent cultural model of illness across cultural/linguistic contexts, with limited shifts in the subtleties of meaning in response to context. Research participants developed a translinguistic biomedical toolkit that they applied in interactions with multiple communities and global health groups. It is in this sense that I develop the concept of transposition.

CHAPTER DESCRIPTIONS

The remainder of the book explores the Thembeka choir's constitution of support and activism at the margins of global health groups and home communities, focusing on their linguistic and cultural practices of HIV transposition across these social contexts. From a broader perspective, the book documents and theorizes how research participants creatively responded to the dynamics of global health interventions in the South African AIDS epidemic. Marginalized in biomedical interventions, aid groups, and home communities, members of the Thembeka choir were able to position them- selves at the intersection of these overlapping groups. This analysis contributes to scholarship at the intersection of linguistic, medical, and psychological anthropology through the development of the concepts of bio-speech com- munity and transposition.

While the chapters in this book may be read individually, they are not designed to be read in such a fashion. Rather, each chapter builds upon and engages with the previous chapters in an attempt to create a coherent argu- ment about language, medicine, and experience over the course of the book. Chapter 2, "Conducting Ethnographic Fieldwork amid Globalized Inequities and Stigma," utilizes a series of ethnographic vignettes to provide readers with more information about the research process as well as historical back- ground, cultural context, and information about the Thembeka choir's begin- nings. I give a brief overview of the history of colonialism and apartheid that shaped racialized inequality in South Africa for readers unfamiliar with this history, as well as a short discussion of the development of the South African AIDS epidemic through the 1990s and early 2000s—the time period when the Thembeka choir was created. This leads to a discussion of how both stigma and socioeconomic marginalization shaped the choir's existence in the world of global health in 2008, after the choir had officially separated from Durban Hospital. I also discuss research methodology, focusing on how HIV stigma impacted ethnographic research methods commonly employed by linguistic anthropologists.

Chapter 3, "The Embodied Reflexivity of a Bio-Speech Community," introduces the choir in the space where group members most often encoun- tered one another—in choir rehearsals. The chapter synthesizes medical anthropology's theorization of biosociality with a close look at embodied communicative practices, focusing especially on performance. In the chap- ter, I discuss two key genres of HIV transposition in the choir's linguistic repertoire, analyzing how Thembeka choir members joked about and sang about HIV. It was in rehearsals that group members were most explicit in their critiques of other South Africans' stigmatizing ways of talking about and conceptualizing HIV. Their reflexive attention to their own and others' lin- guistic practices often occurred in performance-based genres, notably joking and singing. Singing, in particular, was deeply embodied, as vocal cords, lungs, bodies, and minds synchronized with one another to make music in four-part harmony. Here, anthropological theorization of reflexive embodiment provides a key to understanding the role of performance in constructing support, and thus in (re)constituting this bio-speech community through the transposition of HIV.

In chapter 4, "The Power of Global Health Audiences," the focus shifts from how research participants interacted with one another to their encounters with global health professionals. I examine how Thembeka choir members told their stories to such audiences, how their musical performances were shaped by these audiences, and how global health professionals responded to people living with HIV. This analysis is contextualized with discussion of how the transnational circulation of discourses, resources, medication, viruses, and people was shaped by the fault lines of inequality. Drawing from scholarship on audience, recipient design, and the culturally shaped power of listening subjects, I analyze global health audiences as listeners whose social positioning and access to resources impacted how the choir bio-speech community managed global health encounters.

Chapter 5, "HIV Transposition amid the Multiple Explanatory Models of Science, Faith, and Tradition," delves deeper into the ways that the practice of transposition, a central part of the choir bio-speech community's verbal repertoire, intersected with available cultural models of HIV in South Africa. Like other South Africans, group members drew from three models of illness associated with biomedicine, Christian faith, and Zulu tradition. However, choir members explicitly rejected explanations rooted in notions of witchcraft and engaged with faith and tradition in ways that privileged biomedical understandings of HIV/AIDS. They transposed biomedical models into faith-based healing and Zulu traditional medicine. This chapter showcases how the ethnographic approach utilized in this book complements linguistic analysis with an examination of cultural models and explanatory frameworks of illness, revealing a more nuanced and complex management of multiple causal explanations of HIV/AIDS. Group members' transposition of HIV responded both to their positioning at the margins of multiple communities and to the biopower of scientific medicine.

Chapter 6, "The Linguistic Anthropology of Stigma," analyzes the role of linguistic structure and language ideology in both stigma and support. In the chapter, I advance a language-centered theory of stigmatization. Building upon previous research on HIV stigma in South Africa, I discuss how HIV was linguistically marked as foreign and how that foreignness was tied to avoidance and fears of pollution. This includes examination of metalinguistic commentary—persons talking about how others talk about HIV. Stigma and disclosure are two sides of the same coin. Stigma makes disclosure a relevant communicative activity, and the culturally specific contours of stigma are significant in the construction of ideologies of disclosure (e.g., who should disclose, when, if it is valued, and how it is valued). Through the linguistic analysis of HIV stigma, the chapter provides context that is necessary for understanding chapter 7's analysis of disclosure.

In chapter 7, "Performance and the Transposition of a Global Health Ethics of Disclosure," I discuss two distinct and sometimes conflicting moral/ethical discourses about HIV disclosure in South Africa. The two discourses were loosely associated with global health/biomedicine and Zulu tradition, respectively. In the chapter, I detail how Thembeka choir members used performance to transpose a global health perspective on disclosure into contexts of Zulu tradition. Here, I first overview a moral/ethical discourse of disclosure rooted in notions of individual rights and responsibilities. The ability to disclose widely was valued by global health professionals in this discourse. Next, I overview a moral/ethical discourse of disclosure rooted in notions of social duties and respect toward kin. This discourse, associated with choir members' home communities, can be traced back to ideals of Zulu tradition. Drawing on scholarship that models HIV disclosure as fundamentally processual, I showcase an instance in which the choir was able to simultaneously embody both moral/ethical discourses through performance to transpose the global health ideology into the context of a Zulu wedding. More broadly, the chapter demonstrates how the choir drew from a verbal repertoire that centered on HIV transposition to navigate the complexities and dilemmas linked to their positioning at the margins of multiple communities.

The book concludes with a return to the core concepts of bio-speech community and HIV transposition. Here, I review the three traditional requirements of a speech community, discussing how the Thembeka choir's shared verbal repertoire and language ideologies were centered on HIV transposition. Choir members transposed HIV across global health groups and home communities from which they were marginalized. In doing so, they constituted and maintained a bio-speech community—that is, a community oriented toward not only a shared biomedical diagnosis, but also a shared verbal repertoire and language ideologies that shaped how they discussed HIV, conceptualized it, and acted in the context of stigma and global health interventions.

2 · CONDUCTING ETHNOGRAPHIC FIELDWORK AMID GLOBALIZED INEQUITIES AND STIGMA

This chapter provides historical and ethnographic information that helps contextualize the rest of this book. My engagement with South Africa began in earnest in the summer of 2004, when I completed an intensive introductory isiZulu course at Ohio University as part of the Summer Cooperative African Languages Institute. This was followed by participation in a summer intensive isiZulu language and culture program in Pietermaritzburg, South Africa, in 2005 that was funded by the Fulbright-Hays Group Projects Abroad Program, and a short pilot fieldwork visit to Durban in 2006. In 2008, my fieldwork methods included participant-observation of everyday life and social events for research participants, audio-video recording of choir rehearsals and social events, audio-recorded interviews with research participants, audio-recorded interviews conducted by a research assistant (Amahle), and participant-observation at a global health organization, where I attended community advisory board meetings (with several choir members) for a major biomedical HIV treatment study. Finally, I traveled to Durban in 2013 for a brief follow-up visit, and I maintain contact with some research participants on social media. This chapter provides context for the data collected through these processes and the subsequent analysis of the data: context about how HIV was linked to historical inequities in South Africa, about how stigma shaped the research process, and about how the Thembeka choir's marginal connections to global health shaped their group dynamics.

HIV/AIDS IN SOUTH AFRICA'S SOCIOHISTORICAL CONTEXT

HIV/AIDS is a disease of modernity. Often popularly associated with poverty in developing nations, in reality the virus tends to follow the fault lines of inequality and marginalization. The distinction is significant. It is not absolute privation that increases one's chances of being infected with HIV; rather, it is relative privation—a state of inequity in comparison to the wealth of nearby others. The resulting power differentials are sometimes enacted in sexual relationships. In heterosexual encounters in post-apartheid South Africa, as in other patriarchal contexts, this was manifest especially where entrenched gender hierarchies meant that men were the ones who controlled access to limited wealth. Such a pattern resulted in the opportunity for men to have power in sexual relationships: for instance, to refuse condom use, to have multiple girlfriends/sexual partners (either during the same time period or in close succession), or to sexually assault women without penalty or punishment, all of which increased the incidence of HIV infection (Susser 2009).

Inequity is a pervasive feature of the contemporary world economic system, in and beyond South Africa. There, the impact of neoliberalism has further entrenched inequities that developed over hundreds of years of colonialism and apartheid. Apartheid is an Afrikaans word that is literally translated as apartness.[1] The political system of apartheid was inspired by the same eugenics philosophy that shaped segregation in the United States. After over a century of European colonial expansion into southern Africa and conflict between Dutch and British settlers, in 1911 white residents created the Republic of South Africa. Policies that suppressed and oppressed nonwhites, which had already been in place for many years, continued to be expanded. However, the term "apartheid" refers specifically to the post–World War II period from 1948 to 1994 when the National Party was in power. During apartheid, the South African government enacted laws that restricted the movement of, education for, and opportunities available to nonwhites.

One way that this minority government was able to maintain apartheid laws was through violence and physical force. Another way was through a divide-and-conquer policy that separated people into "races." The Population Registration Act of 1950 classified individuals as black (referring to descendants of precontact Africans), Indian (referring to descendants of indentured servants and others who migrated from South Asia), coloured (referring to people of mixed heritage), and white (referring to descendants of precontact Europeans), while the Group Areas Act of 1950 prescribed where people could live according to their race. The black "race" was further divided into discrete ethnic groups—Zulu, Xhosa, Ndebele, Swazi, Bapedi, Basotho, Tswana, Tsonga, and Venda. Both the racial and the ethnic divisions of apartheid ignored a substantial amount of cultural, genetic, and linguistic exchange and attempted to control ambiguity through classificatory rules, forced removals from homes and neighborhoods, and educational segregation. The apartheid government continued a colonial tradition of indirect rule, or "decentralized despotism," by allocating limited authority to traditional leaders, such as the Zulu king (Mamdani 1996). In what is now the province of KwaZulu-Natal, an ethnic Zulu "homeland" (named KwaZulu) was created alongside eight other ethnic homelands, with care taken to ensure that few economic opportunities were available there, while white South Africans maintained control of the most valuable and fertile land (named Natal) (Thompson 2000). The resulting so-called KwaZulu homeland was a fractured conglomeration of close to twenty separate rural areas.

Apartheid distinctions and policies were especially disruptive for the many South Africans who had moved to cities in search of upward mobility prior to the 1940s. Black South Africans whose families had identified as cosmopolitan members of an educated middle class were forcibly cast into tribal and racial molds. In the 1950s, white South African cities were unable to function without cheap labor. As a result, the apartheid government developed the "townships" or "locations" near the cities. These were planned, segregated communities where black, Indian, and coloured workers were forced to live (separate from one another as well as separate from white South Africans). Many informal settlements that included shacks and shebeens (unlicensed bars) also sprung up nearby to support the overflow population that was

working or seeking work. The most famous of these—actually a conglomeration of multiple informal settlements and townships—is named Soweto
("southwest townships"). As the apartheid government enacted ever more
restrictive segregation legislation, they also passed the Bantu Education Act.
This act was meant to prepare black South Africans for the menial jobs they
were expected to take as adults. The law spurred the further development of
the black consciousness movement in South Africa. In 1974, Afrikaans was
made the compulsory language of schooling for black South African children.
Young people mobilized against this development, leading to what might
have been a peaceful protest on June 16, 1976. Instead, police fired tear gas
and then live ammunition at protesters, many of whom were children. One
of the first victims of this tragedy was named Hector Peterson, and his name
became a rallying cry for an uprising that would become national and last
for over a year.

   In Durban, several Thembeka choir members had been raised in the formerly legally segregated township of Umlazi during the last years of apartheid (the mid- to late 1980s). Many family members of township dwellers
remained in the rural homelands, resulting in patterns of circular migration
where workers (often men) lived apart from women in the squalor of impoverished townships, informal settlements, and mining hostels, returning home
occasionally to visit family. Over multiple generations, the racial and ethnic
divisions of colonialism and apartheid, enforced through spatial separation
and differential treatment, became naturalized and shaped not only people's
opportunities but also, in many cases, their perceptions of themselves and
others (Hansen 2012).

   Many members of the choir grew up in Umlazi in the late 1970s and early
1980s amid the brutal violence that characterized the end of apartheid. At that
time, armed insurgence intensified. The apartheid government fomented
conflict between a main antiapartheid organization (panracial in orientation), the African National Congress (ANC), and a Zulu-based political
organization, the Inkatha Freedom Party (IFP). In townships and informal
settlements near Durban, fighting among black South Africans was particularly intense. Despite the fighting, several core group members had lived near
each other in the township and performed in musical groups throughout
their youth.

   In 1994, the first democratic elections were held in South Africa. Under
the leadership of Nelson Mandela and the ANC, the new government focused

on dismantling structural racism, encouraging growth and development in the former homelands and townships, trying to keep the wealth of white South Africans in the country, and convincing foreign investors that South Africa would remain a stable economic powerhouse on the continent. Many have criticized the ANC for pursuing neoliberal economic policies that have led to increasing (racialized) inequities. One of the wealthier nations in Africa, South Africa is now also one of the most unequal countries in the world. Wealth is concentrated in the hands of a very few South Africans of all racial backgrounds, though white South Africans are still much more likely than others to be wealthy. However, neoliberal economic policies were encouraged or required by investors. These policies exacerbated the HIV epidemic by facilitating new forms of circular migration and inequality within South African communities (Hunter 2007). By 2018, the World Bank had named South Africa the country with the highest income inequality in the world.

In the mid-1990s, Nelson Mandela and the ANC knew about the increasing threat of HIV but focused their efforts elsewhere, on issues such as housing for the poor. When the nation's second president, Thabo Mbeki, took over in 1999, the epidemic was in full force. Many members of the Thembeka choir fell ill and received their HIV-positive diagnosis in the late 1990s. Similar to the early days of the U.S. AIDS epidemic, in South Africa fear and stigma had taken hold (Crimp 1987; Treichler 1999). And similar to U.S. president Ronald Reagan's devastating inaction and silence about the epidemic in the 1980s, South African president Thabo Mbeki was at first quiet. He then later embraced fringe scientific views that insisted that the HIV virus was not linked to AIDS (acquired immunodeficiency syndrome). When he might have encouraged testing and open dialogue, Mbeki entrenched himself in what he called "traditional" African values, which included avoidance of talk about sex. His health minister told people to exercise and eat garlic and beetroot to keep their immune system healthy. Mbeki, an antiapartheid activist and freedom fighter, earned a master's degree in economics at Sussex University. His refusal to engage the epidemic was rooted in a thoroughgoing distrust of scientific experts because other "experts" had, in his lifetime, justified apartheid with pseudoscientific eugenics (Fassin 2007). As a result of the government's inaction on HIV, antiretroviral medications (ARVs) were not available to choir members and others in the early 2000s. Infected individuals such as the participants in my research had few options open to them.

People were dying, and hospitals had few tools to treat them. They were sometimes being turned away, told to go home to die (Oppenheimer and Bayer 2007). At this time, a local private hospital, Durban Hospital, opened the doors to its AIDS clinic. Durban Hospital was a Christian-affiliated institution that had been founded by an American missionary in the early twentieth century. In the late 1990s, a choir began there as a women's support group associated with this clinic.

In the early 2000s, a number of choir members became active with the South African Treatment Action Campaign (TAC). The TAC is an HIV/ AIDS activist organization, founded in 1998, that works to counter government inaction and gain patient access to medication and treatment in South Africa's public health system. It would be a mistake, however, to oversimplify the TAC as uniformly positive and President Mbeki's health policy as uniformly negative (Fassin and Schneider 2003). Choir members participated in public protests that eventually led the government to reverse its stance and provide HIV care and access to ARVs beginning in 2004. Despite the "rollout" of ARVs, in 2008 government health care for HIV still entailed long waits for medication. Many group members continued to go to Durban Hospital's HIV clinic for care. The clinic, which had been funded by private donations from South Africans, Americans, and Europeans, and was later supplemented by funding from the U.S. government's PEPFAR initiative, had been providing ARVs at low cost to clinic patients for several years.

The Tenuousness of Legitimacy

Most members of the Thembeka choir were in their mid- to late thirties. As mentioned, several core group members—including Philani, Thulani, Siphesihle, and Fanele, had grown up with each other in the township and performed together in musical groups throughout their youth. After the support group associated with the Durban Hospital AIDS clinic was formed in the late 1990s, women met to talk about their illness experiences and to do South African beadwork together. These beadwork projects were to be sold to help raise money for treatment and to provide a source of income for these women living in poverty. As was common among many isiZulu speakers and other South Africans, the women sang songs as they worked. A hospital social worker suggested that they form a vocal group. Women from the group recruited a few men, including choir leader Thulani, and Thulani encouraged some of his friends who were men to join. In this way, the choir was born.

In 2002, a musician who was part of a U.S.-based Christian aid organization visited Durban and met with the choir. This led to an invitation to travel to the United States on tour to spread awareness and solicit donations for the hospital's AIDS clinic. It also resulted in a feature-length documentary created by two American film students and ethnomusicological fieldwork conducted by another researcher in 2007. By 2008, when I worked with the choir, they had been on tour five times to the United States and Great Britain. The money they raised had helped in the construction of a new building for Durban Hospital's AIDS clinic. Choir members were proud of these accomplishments. However, when I worked with the group they had formally separated from the AIDS clinic. For much of my fieldwork, the details of this separation were fuzzy to me. I eventually learned that members of the choir felt exploited—like they were poster children for an organization but did not receive enough benefits of their work for themselves or others living with HIV. Group members did receive treatment and support, and they gained knowledge about their illness from the hospital. This conflict between the opportunities yielded by association with international aid, on the one hand, and the power dynamic engendered by that association with well-meaning doctors and researchers who nonetheless had relative wealth and power, on the other hand, is central to understanding the choir.

The choir was unique as a musical troupe that was also a support group. At the same time, it was one among many support organizations for people with HIV that developed in the late 1990s and early 2000s. The cultural developments of these illness-oriented groups have been described with the term "biosociality." In southern Africa, biosociality has often been "laid down along already existing networks of family and neighbors, reinforced by shared practices, such as clinic attendance, and the recognition of symptoms in others that have been experienced in one's own body" (Marsland 2012: 473). Indeed, knowledge of the support group had generally been passed by word of mouth among trusted friends and family. Association of support and activist groups with nonprofit organizations and other institutions led to a sense of legitimacy rooted in links with biomedicine (Fassin 2009). By 2008, though, this legitimacy was being threatened by the severing of its relationship with the Durban Hospital AIDS clinic.

ETHNOGRAPHIC METHODS AMID STIGMA

I knew little about this state of the choir's relationship with the hospital when I first arrived in South Africa to conduct fieldwork. It seemed that it was in no one's interest to divulge too much information about this. The separation had the potential to make the hospital look bad and thus endangered continuing grants and donations that funded their treatment and support activities. Meanwhile, a number of choir members worked at the hospital as low-paid lay counselors, and group members returned there as patients for low-cost treatment, so their treatment and income depended on maintaining a good relationship with the hospital. While marginalization from global health groups was a major aspect of the choir's existence (more to come on this), my first few months of ethnographic research were centered around understanding the choir as a community of support and learning how to conduct fieldwork amid stigma.

My First Rehearsal

It is February 17, 2008. I am preparing to observe my first choir rehearsal. I walk from my apartment down a hill through a middle-class Durban neighborhood where I live to a taxi rank where people line up to take minibuses from downtown to places throughout the region.[2] I pack only a small notebook hidden inside an opaque plastic shopping bag. In Durban, it is uncommon for people to carry around backpacks. To do so might arouse unwanted interest in the bag's contents. The minibus taxis—compact vans that squeezed up to seventeen passengers in them—are called kombis, named after a particular model of Volkswagen van produced in the 1950s.

At the taxi rank I meet a choir member, Bongiwe, who would show me the way to their rehearsals. Bongiwe is a woman in her mid-thirties. Her specialty is helping children who were born HIV positive to cope with the virus. She is a large woman and, like many Zulu women raised outside the city, values her size. Born and raised on a farm, Bongiwe considers herself to be a simple woman. She has an earnest way about her that makes me feel at ease. At this point in the research process, I have already met with choir leaders Philani and Thulani and received initial approval to come to a rehearsal. This led to an exchange of emails with Bongiwe, after which I met Bongiwe at Durban Hospital's HIV clinic, where she works as a low-paid lay counselor.

At that time, Bongiwe offered to be my chaperone to the rehearsal because she had to switch taxis at the downtown rank anyway. She traveled far, beginning her journey in a rural informal settlement north of the city that had a reputation for being particularly rough.

Bongiwe describes herself as a very "traditional" woman who never thought of doing anything but staying at home in the rural area and raising a family. After marrying her husband, she stayed in his rural area homestead while he moved to Durban to find work. This was a common practice among people from rural areas. For generations, it had been primarily black South African men who migrated from apartheid "homelands" to cities in search of employment, while the rural homelands became places for women, children, men without work, and men home briefly from work. Recently, more women had begun to also engage in this pattern of movement, termed circular migration. However, Bongiwe did not. She eventually moved to Durban to care for her husband when he fell ill after becoming infected with HIV. Living in a shack with a leaky tarp for a roof, she had gone for testing and discovered she, like her husband, was HIV positive.

Though she rarely speaks about it, Bongiwe had become infected due to her husband's infidelity while away from her, but she stayed with him and cared for him. Her husband recovered from the initial sickness caused by immunodeficiency. The couple saved money and was eventually able to build a four-room cinderblock house that resembled a government-built township home (with two bedrooms, living room, bathroom, and kitchen) topped with a corrugated metal roof. They later added an indoor toilet. Her home was up on a hill overlooking the verdant countryside. The home was inaccessible by car, so Bongiwe had to walk about fifteen minutes to the road, where she would wait for a minibus taxi to drive her to the downtown area, where she would switch taxis to go to the township.

During the week, the downtown taxi rank was always crowded with people waiting in long lines to catch a ride home from the compact downtown area, dominated by tall buildings. On this Sunday, it is the taxis that are waiting in lines to be filled with enough passengers to leave on their journey. When I meet Bongiwe at the taxi rank I have no idea where we are going. I ask her, and she says we are going to one of the townships. Later, some researchers would tell me it was not safe to go to the township at any time of day or night. I am glad I went before I heard this warning. I think that these warnings were as much about racist and/or class-based stereotypes as they were about an increase in danger.

Here is an excerpt from my field notes about the journey and my first impressions of the rehearsal:

The kombi was hot and crowded, and I sat in the very back, squished in between a small girl and a 30-something man. . . . The drive took us on the freeway past the airport, then up into the hills. There were soon shacks by the road, tiny shops in what looked like old train boxcars or harbor freight containers with windows cut out of the side, and many people standing around, waiting for kombis, talking, walking, having a good time. The drive took quite a while. Bongiwe told me that the drive would be faster if we were in our own car, but the kombi wound its way through the community, making stops whenever someone requested it or whenever the driver could attract another passenger with his beeping horn and hand signs. The hand signs, Bongiwe reminded me, were used to distinguish different routes. I'll have to figure those out. We finally got off the kombi and turned onto a smaller road. . . . As we got close to the house where the choir was going to rehearse, Philani drove up with a carload of other choir members.

We entered through the front gate of the house (almost all houses have heavily protective gates and often razor wire to discourage thieves).

I discovered that the rehearsal was going to take place in the garage of the home. It seemed like quite a large home for the area, and in relatively good condition, except for part of a concrete bannister that was missing on a second story balcony. But we never went into the house. After Siphesihle's father (he was introduced as baba meaning "father") pulled a van out of the garage, I looked in to see quite a lot of musical equipment. A PA system and a few amps, a little keyboard and a drum set. It did not look like it was in good condition. This was later confirmed when one of the speakers for the PA system wasn't working. Ndumiso, the drummer, worked on the speaker for quite a while but eventually used another speaker. All in all, there were four women singers, one male singer, a piano player, bass player and a drummer. I guess there have been more people in the past but often not everyone is able to show up (for example, Thulani wasn't there). Some of the women changed from their jeans (street clothes) into other clothes. Celokuhle put on a more traditional South African skirt with some bead designs woven into it; Bongiwe put on some black spandex pants and some black shoes with bead designs woven into them. It seemed to be either for my benefit, or for getting into the feel of rehearsing, or rehearsing the way they would perform.

Stigma and Audio-Video Recording

After that first rehearsal, two months passed in which my weeks were oriented toward Sunday choir practice. When I first began working with the group, I was invited to choir rehearsals and expected to video-record them. It was also acceptable for me to audio-record interviews with group members in private locations. Other than this, my access to research participants' lives was initially limited. When group members first invited me to attend social events, a large part of the motivation to include me seemed to be the services I could provide—for instance, rental car transportation to the funeral described in the introduction, and videography and photography for a wedding. Choir members were friendly, welcoming, and helpful, but cautious about my intrusion into their precarious lives amid stigma. It was only after I demonstrated my ability to "blend in," as Fanele later explained it, by displaying my understanding of some of the social complexities of living with HIV, that I was included in more mundane social activities where subtlety, indirection, or silence on the topic of HIV was needed.

One challenge of linguistic anthropological fieldwork in this context was learning how to utilize audio-video recording in ways that responded to research participants' acts of disclosure and nondisclosure. Linguistic anthropologists tend to try and record anything and everything that research participants say, because we never know when a social encounter might provide significant insight into links between language and culture. While cultural and medical anthropologists utilize audio-video recording technologies to a lesser extent, the use of video and audio is becoming more common in those subfields as recording technologies become more ubiquitous. Audio-video recording drew attention to research participants and yielded questions from non–group members about my intentions and research focus that were sometimes unwelcome, because these questions threatened research participants' nondisclosure. My decisions about when and how to record thus also became a display to research participants of my understanding of the cultural conventions about HIV disclosure. My ability to use technology with respect (*hlonipha*) during fieldwork led group members to open up to me and incorporate me into their broader social networks (including family members, neighbors, and friends). As fieldwork progressed, I learned that sometimes having a recorder at hand but not using it was an indication of respect and understanding.

One space where I was able to demonstrate my sensitivity to group members' communicative and social needs was during car rides to and from rehearsals. As mentioned, when I first attended choir rehearsals I traveled by minibus taxi. Later, I switched to a long-term car rental. In doing so, I was also able to offer choir members increased safety and decreased costs associated with traveling to rehearsals. Every Sunday, I drove into downtown Durban to pick up group members Bongiwe, Dumisile, and Sthembile, all of whom were commuting to rehearsals from outside the township. The downtown pickup was stressful for all research participants. The taxi rank was not a safe place for them to hang around, especially not on Sundays when fewer people were there, and timing our various arrivals was always tricky. Research participants' difficulties regarding safety and travel were part and parcel of the very same inequities that shaped patterns of HIV infection and marginalization in global health.

The car rides to rehearsals became one of the few spaces outside of rehearsals where group members could talk freely about HIV without fear of being overheard by others, such as family, friends, or random strangers. I soon noticed that Bongiwe, Dumisile, and Sthembile (along with others who sporadically came to rehearsals) would talk about anything and everything related to HIV in the car—for instance, a staph infection associated with reduced immune system response, the issue of disclosing to a new boyfriend, and questions about how to talk to a son about his HIV infection (he had been born with HIV) when he was getting old enough to ask questions about why he took medication.

These were important, revealing conversations that might have made excellent recorded data for my project. On several occasions I had my audio recorder ready in the car with the intent to ask for permission to use it during our rides to and from rehearsals, but my intuitions about the impact of doing so led me to keep the recorder off and out of the way. Utilizing the recorder would have meant introducing new (imagined) listeners, in the form of scholars, students, and any others who might read about my research or see it presented in the future. To do so would have cut off this new space for support. Soon, others began to ask me if I could drive them places. Over the next few months, I crisscrossed the province of KwaZulu-Natal with choir members going to weddings, funerals, birthday parties, and other social events. This was of mutual advantage to all of us, since my research directly benefited from being included in these activities. I never used a recorder while in the car. Here, the recorder was not just absent, it was noticeably absent. Group members saw when I turned on the audio recorder or video camera. They also attended to when I did not. Having these technologies available but not using them communicated to group members that I understood the dynamics of stigma, support, and respect (*hlonipha*).

Audio-video recorders became an extension of my social self. I could display myself as a moral/ethical entity who understood that group members benefited from a safe space (the car) in which they could be free from worries about disclosure that they usually negotiated in the context of pervasive HIV stigma. I was, of course, listening, but the capacity of the recorder to reproduce a given conversation in full represented a different sort of listening and documentation that was more complete, less anonymous, and more intrusive. In the case of car rides with research participants, I utilized the disconnect between my own observation and that of the recorder to present myself as a social being who was sensitive to the exigencies of stigma.

CHALLENGES OF LOCALIZING GLOBAL HEALTH ACTIVISM

It may seem incongruous that the choir could be a performance group and activist organization but could also be worried about disclosure of members' HIV-positive status. In fact, there were several different ways that the choir managed disclosure for different audiences. Group members took advantage of the stark social divide between global health audiences that were mostly middle class, white, and/or international, on the one hand, and other audiences consisting of neighbors, friends, and families. When they performed at global health events, the choir could be announced as an HIV-positive choir; yet in the township they could still be known to most as a performance troupe. After officially separating from Durban Hospital, the choir struggled to create a new vision that would enable them to access the resources of global health, engage in activism, and yet still be sensitive to the need of some individual choir members to avoid disclosure in township contexts. Alongside these challenges presented by HIV stigma, choir activist activities were also limited by a lack of training in bureaucratic skills needed to obtain global health grants and donations without using the hospital as an intermediary.

A Youth Day Speech

Such challenges and limitations were evident at a children's choir competition in the township that the Thembeka choir organized in June 2008. They planned the competition to fall on a weekend when they could celebrate both Father's Day and Youth Day. Youth Day is a South African holiday that commemorates the Soweto Uprising of 1976. Some choir members had been acting as directors and teachers for a neighborhood girls' choir primarily composed of AIDS orphans. This was one of a number of activist projects that individual group members were spearheading. I attended some of the girls' choir rehearsals, but I did not include this activity as data for my project because I did not have IRB approval to conduct research with children. While I describe the public Father's Day/Youth Day celebration and youth choir competition in the following pages, my focus remains on Thembeka choir members' actions for this same reason.

On the day of the competition, I arrive at a community center near where the Thembeka choir normally rehearses. Folding chairs are lined up in rows facing a stage where the choir's instruments and sound equipment are set up. I record over five hours of video and later share this with choir members so that the children can have a record of their performances. In the process, I also record two speeches—one made by Fanele in honor of Youth Day and one made by Philani in honor of Father's Day. When it is time for Fanele to give her speech, she approaches the microphone on stage and begins (in isiZulu):

> My heart is grieving. I want you to hear me. My heart is grieving when a parent does not take action, because it wasn't their child's blood by which today we are free. If mine could have been taken—[Fanele's child's name] who is the same age as Hector Peterson—to be shot so that your child should enjoy life, that would have been painful to me. My heart grieves when children do not have knowledge of what was happening. About what was happening . . . we will not go to school tomorrow. It is necessary that we teach about who died, parents. It is necessary that we teach. Children, do you hear my tears?

The children in the audience respond in unison, *"yebo* (yes)." Fanele seems to be upset that not enough children know about the Soweto Uprising, that they just celebrate Youth Day as an excuse to not go to school. But she is also speaking to the few parents who are in the audience, preparing them to see a parallel between the events of the Soweto Uprising and the current devastation of the AIDS pandemic.

After the children respond, Fanele continues (in isiZulu, translation below with English code-mixing in bold):

> *Ngoba nibona izingane zilana namhlanje kuyafana esibhekene nakho*
> Because you see, children, being here today, what we are coming across is similar

> *nokwakubhekene nezingane zika **nineteen seventy six**. Namhlanje elethu igazi*
> to the children of **1976**. Today our blood

> *liphalala, lithathwe i **HIV**. Nginamanga yini?*
> is overflowing, being taken by **HIV**. Am I lying?

In Fanele's subsequent four-minute speech, "HIV" is notable as one of only a few English words (the number "1976" is also in English—choir members and others living in the township often used English to refer to dates and numbers). As my research progresses, I learn that this use of English for HIV reference is a notable pattern in choir members' linguistic practices. Fanele goes on with her speech, emphasizing the importance of parents talking to their children about sex and HIV and the importance of supporting their children. She explains that she and the other choir members are acting as "role models" in "mentorship" roles with a girls' choir (borrowing these English words), and she asks parents to do the same. Neither Fanele nor any of the other choir members disclose that they are a choir made up of people living with HIV.

Fanele continues to discuss parental involvement throughout her Youth Day speech, ending by comparing HIV with other wars and battles (in isiZulu, with the English translation below each line and English words in bold):

> *Bantakwethu, siba **supporte**, sibasekele ngayo yonke indlela,*
> My dears, we must **support** them, we must prop them up by all means,

sibavumele, basichazele ukuthi kwenziwani, sibambisaneni njengabazali
we must agree with them, they must explain to us what they are doing, we must
work together as parents

neyingane ukuze ikusasa lethu liphephe empini esilwa nayo namhlanje,
with the child, so that our tomorrow is saved in the war we are battling today—

izidakamizwa, i HIV, ubudlova, yonke lento eyenza ukuthi izingane zethu
substance abuse, **HIV**, rioting, all these things from which our children

zingakhululeki nakuba ziphila ezweni elikhululekile. Ngiyanibonga ke.
are not free, even though they are living in a free world. I thank you, then.

The idea that HIV was something to be fought had become a common trope
in South African public discourse (and in globally circulating discourses
about HIV/AIDS). This way of mobilizing people had particularly poignant
undertones in the historical context of previous battles against apartheid.
Indeed, some people talked about AIDS as "the new apartheid." In her Youth
Day speech, Fanele took this metaphor one step further, using the memory
of the Soweto Uprising as an opportunity to engage in activism. Throughout her speech she spoke almost exclusively in isiZulu except when using
English terms related to HIV/AIDS. She never used the isiZulu terms *isifo
sofuba* (sickness of the chest—TB) or *ingculazi* (AIDS), and she never used
stigmatizing terms, such as *i slim* (slim) or *iqhoks* (high-heeled shoes), but
rather transposed valued scientific medical and psychological terminology
(such as *i HIV* and *i support*) into her isiZulu Youth Day speech.

While this Youth Day event was a success, it nonetheless demonstrated
some of the challenges that Thembeka choir members faced at the borders of
global health networks and home communities. Their ability to engage in HIV
activism in this space was shaped by the need of some group members to maintain anonymity in home communities due to the threat of stigma. Interconnected with stigma was the dominant cultural convention of speaking to elders
with respect, which further limited the sorts of topics that Fanele and others
could address. Finally, leaders such as Fanele could only speak in generalities
about HIV prevention while avoiding the disclosure of the choir's function as
an HIV support group. In these ways, HIV stigma and Zulu tradition limited
the possibility of localizing the Thembeka choir's activist activities.

Receipts and Responsibilities

Though Thembeka choir members and other Zulu AIDS activists were able to productively exploit their position at the boundaries of the overlapping groups of global health, creatively facing stigma and constituting support through their engagement with biomedicine, their actions were simultaneously limited by their positioning at the margins of these groups. The youth choir competition is just one example of the sort of event that Thembeka choir members thought would be effective as an HIV-prevention activity. One group member worked with a girls' netball team and a boys' soccer team. Another had the idea of buying a van so that the choir could travel to schools to perform and provide information about HIV/AIDS to Durban-area children. Choir members tried to enact policies and organize activities that they knew were associated with global health granting activities, but lacked the training, and most significantly, the credentials needed to directly access funding. Still, the choir made efforts to engage with global health through adoption of bureaucratic practices throughout 2008. One encounter in particular provided a clear example of these efforts.

It is early March 2008, at the end of the first choir rehearsal that I have video-recorded. Choir members form a circle to hold a group meeting (other topics discussed during this meeting are detailed in other chapters). Among other things, this meeting includes a focus on the choir's bookkeeping practices. The group started a bank account with the small earnings collected through previous paid performances and a check from Durban Hospital that was meant to compensate the choir for a CD they had recorded for the hospital. Celokuhle has been chosen to be their business manager. A lengthy exchange begins, focusing on a donation check that Durban Hospital clinic—where Celokuhle works as a low-paid lay counselor—is supposed to be sending to the choir. The group has waited for weeks and not received any notice from the hospital. Choir members spend several minutes going over the problem and working out what should be done to diplomatically approach hospital staff. Even though the choir is no longer technically affiliated with the hospital, doctors and researchers who are linked to the hospital still act as gatekeepers to various opportunities.

As the discussion about the donation ends, Celokuhle uses the exchange about finances as a springboard to ask several of the men of the group to give her a receipt for an electric keyboard they recently bought with choir funds.

Celokuhle requests (in isiZulu—English code-mixing indicated in bold), "You all (please) bring the **receipt** for the **keyboard** on Sunday."

In response, Philani asks, "What will you do with the **receipts**? I'm just asking."

"We must have a **file** which has **receipts** with everything that we use as a **choir** for the **records**," Celokuhle replies. Her insistence might have been interpreted as merely an interest in organizational bookkeeping. However, Philani's next conversational move shifts the meaning of the request away from bookkeeping toward questions of responsibility, trust, and blame. He suggests that people should give her the receipts, but that Celokuhle should also merely do what she is "responsible for" ("o **responsible** kuyona") and should stop being so intense about people failing to provide receipts.

However, Celokuhle rejects Philani's deflection from her original request, and insists, "Do we not have the right to know about things like those, Philani?"

It would be a mistake, given choir member multilingualism, to interpret every instance of English code-mixing as an index of global health and HIV activism. Still, it is notable that in this exchange, the only English terms that appear are those associated with global health activities and ideologies: "receipt," "keyboard," "file," "choir," "records," and the morally weighted "responsible." Over the next few minutes, several choir members voice concerns about the rigidity with which Celokuhle is suggesting they comply with bureaucratic ideals. The conversation ends without resolution.

Underlying this discussion was constant worry about money and resources, especially worry about whether or not some group members were unfairly benefiting from contact with global health circulation at the expense of others. This was a topic that repeatedly arose during fieldwork. Also, in other conversation during the group meeting, Bongiwe had raised another similar concern. The undercurrent of worry, concern, and allegation was linked to the discussion of bookkeeping practices—practices that were valued by global health—in two ways. First, there was a general scarcity of resources for people living in poverty amid stigma, in conjunction with the relative wealth of global health professionals. This provided a ripe context for possible exploitation and unfair individual gain by group members who made personal friendships with those professionals, while bookkeeping provided a potential check on these possibilities (more to come on this). Second, bookkeeping was seen as a prerequisite for avoiding Durban Hospital

01 Good day, Steve. It's been a long time since we saw or heard from you. I hope
02 you are well. Some of the choir members met last weekend because we are
03 concerned about something. I'm sure you remember the documentary ([Name
04 of Documentary]) that we have. We feel that we should have been paid for it
05 and also we would like to know what is happening with its copies so as the
06 proceeds from the sales if it is being sold. We are concerned about this
07 because this documentary was not the first and we know that we were paid for
08 it even though the money didn't reach us. As I said that some of us, not
09 everybody is in this because we suspect that the money was paid and some
10 people kept it for themselves. These are the people that were in the meeting:
11 Siphesihle, Thulani, Zethu, Gigi, Amahle, Wendy, Sthembile, Bongiwe, and
12 myself. Bongiwe, Gigi, and I were appointed to write to you because we have
13 access to the computer. We decided to have a caucus meeting first, try to
14 gather as much information as possible, then act on it. We agreed that you are
15 the right person to ask to help us get to the bottom of this. Could you please
16 slot our concern into your busy schedule.
17 Thanking you in advance. Here are our contact numbers should you need to
18 call. [Lists phone numbers].
          Best regards
          Celokuhle

FIGURE 2.1. Transcript: We Suspect the Money Was Paid (email 2-1-2013).

as a go-between and instead directly engaging with global health nonprofit organizations and government programs.

Fears of Uneven Distribution of Scarce Resources

These concerns about where money was ending up and whether choir members were treating one another fairly reemerged in early 2013. In this instance, my involvement starts with Celokuhle sending me an email from the Gmail account I helped her to create in 2008. In the email (reproduced in figure 2.1), she asks if I would investigate the current status of a student-made documentary about the choir.

A number of things stand out to me when I read this email. There is implicit chiding and criticism, "It's been a long time since we saw or heard from you" (line 01). This is not entirely fair, I think, since I have been in contact via phone and email with Amahle and Zethu, and via Facebook with Siphesihle and Philani. Still, the implication is that as an American researcher, I am expected to have the financial and technological means to stay in better touch than I have. I am expected to be able to move both digitally and physically across boundaries. In line 07, Celokuhle mentions, "this documentary was not the first." If they are going to be appearing in these sorts of artistic endeavors, choir members think they should be compensated. They also want to know where the money is going, if not to them (lines 07–08). In lines 12–13, Celokuhle mentions that not everyone has access to a computer. In other words, group members have limited access to resources that would enable them to communicate on a global scale or to do their own research into what is happening with the documentary.

Implicit in this email is the fact that some choir members are concerned that other group members are secretly benefiting from the sale of the student-made documentary. This is very similar to an accusation levied against some group members early on in 2008. It is also similar to fears that choir members had articulated that they were being exploited by Durban Hospital clinic. There is a pattern here: repeatedly, choir members are concerned that some persons (either some choir members or other South Africans associated with global health) have unfair access to limited resources as a result of their connections to international donors and researchers.

After Celokuhle's initial query, we send a series of emails back and forth. I learn that the choir's bank account had been closed due to lack of activity. Then I ask about contacting people at the clinic: "Hi Celokuhle, I have tried to find contact info for Scott and Kyle without success. I can try to contact others, like Laura [of TB Leaders] or people at Durban Hospital clinic. But I want to get your approval before I take that step. Steve" Celokuhle responds, "The . . . clinic was closed last year in June so nobody will be able to assist you." After this dead end, I am unable to find any contact information for the documentary's American producers, so the investigation ends here. However, as a result of our exchange, I become concerned about the new problem of Durban Hospital's closure. In addition to receiving medical care there, numerous choir members work as HIV counselors at the hospital. Its closure would mean an end to that meager source of income.

A few weeks after my email exchange with Celokuhle, I am awarded a grant from Georgia State University that will fund a return trip to Durban in the summer of 2013 for follow-up fieldwork. After I arrive in Durban, I learn that though the clinic is indeed closed, the hospital has not yet closed. Some individuals continue to go to the hospital to pick up their ARVs.

At the *braai* (barbecue—a South African word for an event centered around grilling meat) I attend with choir members while in Durban, some group leaders are notably absent. I learn that Fanele and Philani have been ostracized from the group as a result of the accusations hinted at by Celokuhle. I also think that perhaps their recent marriage to one another has played a part in their exclusion—Fanele had previously been in a partnership with Thulani, who is present at the braai. The choir has even excluded Fanele and Philani from a text messaging group on a platform similar to WhatsApp that they have created.

This social maneuvering and scandal were linked to the long-term impacts of the group's marginal positioning at the edges of global health. On a personal level, it was sad to see good friends torn apart by such forces. Taking a step back, though, it was clear that difficulties in the management of social life and in accessing hospital services were part and parcel of the choir's limited connection to the uneven global circulation of resources, people, and communication associated with global health. Though dismissed by some (including a former white South African choir manager) as just conspiracy theories, the content of choir members' stories about exploitation revealed an astute analysis of the movement of resources and people associated with the AIDS pandemic and an accurate portrayal of group members' limited access to that circulation despite their involvement in multiple global health efforts.

CONCLUSION

The Thembeka choir found a space for HIV support and AIDS activism amid stigma at the margins of global health. Performance, in speech and song, was integral in the group's activities of support and activism. Vocal performance also provided a point of connection to the world of global health. The Thembeka choir was valued by global health professionals primarily as a performance troupe. They were a vibrant success story, an auditory and visual reminder of the positive outcomes that were possible through biomedical intervention. Furthermore, the choir's embodiment of activist personas and Christian faith appealed to wealthy donors and doctors alike. However, the group was constrained both by HIV stigma and by their limited ability to connect with the circulation of resources associated with global health.

Certain facets of the choir, such as their reliance on performance in processes of support and activism, were clear to many, including researchers, doctors, and student filmmakers who had worked with the choir before me. However, developing an understanding of other aspects of the group's linguistic and cultural practices, such as the role of embodied reflexivity in the constitution of support, or the ways that global health audiences implicitly shaped choir members' performances and other communication, required my involvement in group members' everyday lives over a period of many months—an involvement that is a central part of ethnographic research methods. HIV stigma presented one set of challenges for the deployment of ethnographic research methods. Participating, observing, and recording in group members' everyday life were only possible after research participants saw that I was beginning to understand the complex navigation of disclosure/ nondisclosure across audience contexts. Globalized, historically shaped inequities presented another set of challenges. Choir members' access to resources associated with global health depended on the good will of doctors and researchers who acted as gatekeepers. Research participants revealed their attitudes about their relationship with these gatekeepers only after they were confident that I was not going to endanger their access to resources by intentionally or unintentionally sharing this privileged information with my global health peers. I feel comfortable sharing this information now, because over ten years have passed, the choir no longer performs, and choir members have moved on to other jobs. As a result, I do not think that my sharing of this anonymized information would endanger future opportunities for group members. Through ethnographic fieldwork, I learned about the role of language and performance in the formation of this unique community but also about the significance of HIV transpositions in the choir's navigation of the borders of global health and home communities.

3 · THE EMBODIED REFLEXIVITY OF A BIO-SPEECH COMMUNITY

On April 1, 2008, about two months into my fieldwork, I go to the township to meet Zethu and help her with her demography homework. I am supposed to meet her at her house (where she lives with Amahle and other family members). Zethu is taking a number of classes through UNISA, a South African university that operates primarily through correspondence. This means that most of the course is to be completed in workbooks and submitted assignments, with no lectures and only a few opportunities to meet with instructors. Correspondence makes the courses cheaper, but much more difficult, especially for individuals for whom English is not their first language. Zethu has asked me if I could help her with her homework, and I have agreed. This is a chance to help someone in the choir and a chance to get to know Zethu better.

At this point in my fieldwork I am still traveling by kombi (minibus taxi) most of the time, renting a car only on the weekends to help group members travel to and from rehearsals and transport my recording equipment and my saxophone. When I get off the kombi in the township neighborhood, Zethu is waiting for me. On our walk to her home, Zethu calmly remarks, "Thulani SMS-ed [texted] me to say that Siphesihle is dead." I do not know what to say. Zethu seems so calm, almost happy. I ask her how he died—maybe in a car accident, or in a shooting? I am worried about bringing up

HIV, thinking that this will peg me as a prejudiced individual. Siphesihle could have died due to any number of causes, I remind myself. This is terrible news.

All of a sudden, Zethu starts laughing uncontrollably. "No," she explains, "sometimes we do this to each other, as a joke." Then she reminds me that it is April Fools' Day. This is an example of a genre of joking in which choir members played with their shared knowledge of each other's HIV-positive status. Along with song, joking was a key genre through which choir members faced HIV stigma.

This chapter explores the role of embodied reflexivity, through language and music, in the communicative formation of the choir as a biosocial group—that is, as a bio-speech community. The chapter focuses especially on two genres of communication that were part of the speech community's shared verbal repertoire—joking about and singing about HIV—and the role of embodied reflexivity as a biosocial response to stigma in these genres. As mentioned in chapter 1, the concept of biosociality is derived from philosopher Michel Foucault's (1965 [1961], 1978, 1979) discussion of biopower and subjectivity. Critically evaluating medicine and psychiatry, Foucault suggests that the medical clinic is a modern institution that asserts power through a discourse of biological innateness. In doing so, biomedicine crafts culturally and historically specific forms of subjectivity that are valued in dominant discourses—biopower. This notion has been incorporated into anthropological examination of how scientific knowledge of the human body may lead to a new sort of biopower, the power to not only understand but also alter genetics and physiology (Rabinow 1992). As people engage more substantively with advances in biomedicine, they may form social groups centered around biogenetic characteristics. For instance, those with a biogenetic tendency toward type 2 diabetes might form a support group to help regulate their eating habits. Indeed, more recent scholarship in medical anthropology discusses how communities form and maintain legitimacy around such biogenetic and biomedical characteristics (e.g., Fassin 2009; Guell 2011; Marsland 2012). This sort of community formation is only one of many options available to sufferers, albeit a heavily privileged and legitimated option in contemporary biomedical contexts (Rapp 1999: 302–303; Whyte 2009).

In such Foucaultian analytic approaches, the term "discourses" usually describes cultural-historical patterns that shape how people could or might speak rather than actual instances of people speaking. However, my analysis of the Thembeka choir's actions, experiences, and long-term development suggest that not only the generalities of "discourses" but also the specifics of how people communicate in particular moments are central to the differentiated constitution of biosocial groups. To model the role of language in these group-formation processes, in this chapter I synthesize the concept of biosociality with linguistic and psychological anthropological approaches to embodiment and reflexivity. I suggest that the choir's prominent use of song and their playful engagement with one another through joking helped the group to be able to communicate about HIV despite stigmatization, and thus to support one another and work as activists within the uneven global circulation of resources and people associated with global health and humanitarian aid. The organization of embodied reflexivity in these two genres of performance enabled the constitution of a community of HIV support and activism—a bio-speech community.

THE SEMIOTIC ORGANIZATION OF EMBODIED REFLEXIVITY

A key goal of the Thembeka choir was to provide support. Many choir members emphasized that the physiological work of singing—of moving bodies together in synchrony, practicing choreographed kicks and other moves—made them feel good. It was a welcome respite from the stresses of their week. As discussed in other research on HIV in South Africa, music provided a way for people to communicate about things that they did not feel able to talk about (McNeill 2011: 155). It was also central to the constitution of biosociality. In other words, music was central in the constitution of support and played a primary role in holding this community together. Choir rehearsals were held each Sunday in a dusty two-car garage next to pianist Siphesihle's house in Umlazi township. Before the group began to make music together, choir members would sweep the floor; move benches, speakers, a keyboard, and a drum set; and make room for the twelve or so regular attendees. At the time of fieldwork, Siphesihle was in his thirties, living in his parents' home with his own children. Though his children may have had a relationship with their mother, I never met her or saw her at the home. Siphesihle's children, along with his nephews and nieces, often drifted through the garage or were called upon to run errands, such as filling a plastic pitcher with water. His brother was also often present, a man living with HIV who had little musical talent but great enthusiasm for the choir and the feeling of support that it generated. Set in this small space that felt insulated from the outside world, rehearsals were often playful. This is something that I was not prepared for. I am not sure what I expected—I suppose I thought that an HIV support group and AIDS activist organization would be focused on somber reflection. What I found was, indeed, reflection, but reflection embedded in a world of vibrant dance, Christian prayer, song, and laughter.

Siphesihle was very thin. He loved to play and joke, and he was also passionate about the study of music. He had grown up living mostly in the township along with other choir members Fanele, Thulani, and Philani. As I got to know him better, Siphesihle often teased me about my isiZulu competence in front of the other choir members, especially when my video camera was on, but it was always lighthearted. He was close friends with Philani, who was also quite thin. Philani was always impeccably dressed and polite but liked to get a little bit boisterous with Siphesihle. One day, they showed me a picture of the two of them from a few years back. In the picture, they posed with their shirts off, flexing their muscles. They had been body builders, but HIV had taken that away from them. As the virus—sometimes referred to as "slim" in stigmatizing discourses—altered their bodies, so too did music and collaborative humor engage their bodies, framing the bodily movement and embodied rhythmic entrainment of performance as part of HIV support and AIDS activism.

While the concept of embodiment is utilized across anthropological subfields in diverse ways, one theme that is shared across distinct scholarly viewpoints is the idea that mind, body, language, and society can and should be understood as holistically integrated with one another. In linguistic anthropology, discussion of embodiment places the analysis of grammar and lexicon in the context of the deployment of other semiotic resources, such as gesture, facial expression, prosody, eye gaze, and body orientation (Streeck et al. 2012). In research on music and language, a focus on sound and the voice details how extrasymbolic meaning-making occurs in the midst of performance (Turino 1999). In medical anthropology, the body is theorized as simultaneously individual, social, and political (Inhorn and Wentzell 2011; Scheper-Hughes and Lock 1987). And in psychological anthropology, scholars conceptualize the body as simultaneously involved in both representation and being-in-the-world (Csordas 1994). Synthesizing these perspectives, this book adds an analysis of performance "on stage" and in everyday life, examining the role of reflexivity in embodied performance. Here, I analyze embodied reflexivity in two pervasive genres of performance through which choir members communicated about HIV: joking about HIV and singing about HIV. This analysis indicates that the intermediate level of embodied reflexivity associated with these two genres functioned to allow participants to face HIV stigma without explicitly talking about HIV. This process played a primary role in the creation and maintenance of the choir as a biosocial community—in other words, as a bio-speech community.

Joking: On the Continuum of Reflexivity

Thembeka choir members sometimes joked around with each other as they waited to start rehearsals. For instance, the following example of joking about HIV occurred as choir members were organizing the garage to prepare for rehearsal in the ways described earlier. On this day, I was helping group members to set up sound equipment for rehearsal. I had turned on my camera and left it on a tripod, recording conversation and activities as we worked. Bongiwe was there early with me, along with choir member Dumisile (a woman). Bongiwe was sweeping the floor and moving a bench out of the way. The choir's drummer, Ndumiso, and bass player, Philani (both men), were also present. Ndumiso lived nearby in a small metal shack in an informal settlement, and Philani was often around with his close friend Siphesihle (in whose garage the rehearsals were held).

In this example, I use a transcript to represent the temporal unfolding of a playful improvisational encounter. A translation is provided in italics below the original to demonstrate the transposition of English medical terms into the joke, with English borrowing/code-mixing in bold. Double parentheses indicate additional information needed to understand the transcript. Throughout the book more generally, I utilize transcripts and descriptions of recorded spoken/sung encounters in ways that are similar to the ways that cultural anthropologists often use ethnographic vignettes. They are chosen as moments that were representative of patterns observed throughout ethnographic fieldwork. For instance, the transcript presented in figure 3.1 represents just one of many times that choir members joked about HIV—some of those moments were audio-video recorded and others were recorded in field notes.

01 Bongiwe:	*sima lapha vele?* ((sweeping and moving a bench)) is it ((the bench)) supposed to be here?
02 Ndumiso:	*yah sima lapha. noma uzosidonsa uhambe naso.* Yeah, it's supposed to be here. or you'll drag it and go (home) with it.
03 Bongiwe:	*hhayibo. ngiyaphuquza mina.* Hey no. Me, I'm making dust.
04 Ndumiso:	*sizoba ne* **TB**. We will get **TB**.
05 Bongiwe:	*kade ngingashaneli bengini phathisa ngethi- ehh. nge* **TB**. I wasn't sweeping I was just infecting you with- ehh. with **TB**.
06 Ndumiso:	mmm.

FIGURE 3.1. Transcript: Making Dust (05-11-2008 tape 1, 11 min 12 sec).

It is May 2008, and I am assisting group members in preparing Siphesihle's garage for choir rehearsal. As she sweeps the garage, Bongiwe asks Ndumiso if a nearby bench is supposed to be where it is. Ndumiso responds playfully, exaggerating that Bongiwe might drag the bench home with her if she moves it. Bongiwe responds in kind, explaining that she is not sweeping but rather making dust. This implies that she might cause harmful dust to move about the room—in traditional Zulu understandings of illness, the movement of air and dust may result in a variety of ailments. Ndumiso then shifts the focus, claiming that they will get tuberculosis (TB), playing on both the traditional Zulu understanding introduced by Bongiwe and the biomedical understanding of pulmonary TB (that TB is transmitted through the air). Bongiwe builds upon that statement, asserting that she is infecting Ndumiso with TB. Ndumiso closes the joke and play frame with the minimal evaluation, "mmm."

Jokes are often difficult to translate, in part because so much content of a joke is culturally specific and in part because so much of a joke remains implicit. The humor in this and the next example is rooted in the transposition of biomedical models of HIV and TB into choir rehearsal contexts. It is significant that Ndumiso and Bongiwe use the English "TB" rather than the isiZulu *isifo sofuba* (literally, illness of the lungs) to describe the infection Bongiwe is supposedly enabling through her sweeping. The isiZulu term would have more narrowly indexed traditional Zulu understandings. Indeed, *isifo sofuba* may refer to a broad swath of illnesses related to breathing and lungs. Many group members considered traditional Zulu understandings of *isifo sofuba* to be superstitious. Instead, Bongiwe and Ndumiso transpose the biomedical conceptualization of TB into their isiZulu conversation through code-mixing/borrowing. This creates a potential incongruence between his use of the English "TB," which indexes a biomedical model, and the discussion of dust, which plays with the Zulu traditional medicine model of becoming sick from breaking dust.

Also, in this excerpt no one mentions HIV outright. Instead, the connection is implicit, embedded within what has been termed a secondary text of the joke. In my experience more generally, Thembeka choir members' joking never addressed HIV directly. Rather, shared knowledge about the virus, and the shared knowledge that everyone in the choir was HIV positive, remained implicit. This knowledge was part of the secondary text of joking, information that is usually understood and laughed about but not commented upon (Basso 1979). Puns provide a simple, if groan-worthy, demonstration of what is meant by a secondary text. For instance, "I was struggling to figure out how lightning works. Then, it struck me." Here, there are two meanings of "struck": the first, linked to the subject of lightning, indicates that the speaker was struck by lightning; the second, linked to the subject of thinking about a difficult problem or puzzle, indicates that the speaker suddenly realized how lightning works. This semantic ambiguity, which is exploited in punning, is an inherent aspect of all languages (Samuels 2004). However, puns and jokes draw attention to it (Sherzer 2002). Joking thus invokes reflexivity.

TB is an opportunistic infection common among South Africans living with HIV, common enough that many people associate the two illnesses and sometimes use the term "TB" to refer to HIV. Here the secondary text includes these ideas: (1) the two participants are living with HIV; (2) they are thus more susceptible to TB infection; and (3) they accept their statuses and thus are willing to play with their biomedical knowledge of HIV/TB co-infection. The collaborative, improvisational co-construction of this joke meant that neither speaker was wholly responsible for the content of the joke. In the context of HIV stigma, the diffusion of responsibility for discussion, even when indirect, about HIV may have contributed to the ability of choir members to be able to broach the topic.

As Ndumiso and Bongiwe collaboratively built this joke, then, they reflected upon and implicitly pointed toward their understandings of traditional Zulu models of illness, biomedical models of illness, the links between

TB and HIV, and their own HIV-positive statuses. Phenomenologically oriented research suggests that such reflexivity is not an all-or-nothing phenomenon. Rather, there is a continuum of experience from the prereflective everyday engagement with the world, on the one hand, to fully articulated reflection on that engagement (e.g., in narrative), on the other (Desjarlais and Throop 2011; Throop 2002). Whether on stage or in everyday life, performance invokes at least some reflexivity as performers and audience members attend to not only the content but also the form of a performance (e.g., the style, poetic devices employed, "stage presence") (Berger and Del Negro 2002). Meanwhile, the framing of communication as performance alters its meaning (e.g., framing the performance as a joke, a ritual invocation, or a fairy tale). Jokes, with their implicit secondary texts, tend to be associated with an intermediate level of reflection. After all, to explain a joke is to ruin it.

The fact that the reflexivity of Ndumiso and Bongiwe's joking remained implicit (and perhaps only partially subject to the speakers' awareness) was likely helpful in allowing the two of them, and other choir members in other instances, to face stigma without discussing it outright. The embodiment of this reflexive transposition of biomedical models was evident in the ways that the two deployed and discussed not only their bodies (sweeping, inhaling or being exposed to pathogens) but also the built environment (the bench, the broom, the garage) (see Goodwin and Goodwin 2000). This brief moment of joking about HIV, similar to others I recorded on camera and in field notes, provides a window into how moments of biosociality emerged in everyday encounters. The embodied reflexivity of such everyday performances helped choir members to create and maintain a bio-speech community oriented toward support and activism.

Infected Again

A second example of choir members' pattern of joking about HIV comes from the very first choir rehearsal that I recorded. As in other instances, this example is highly collaborative and improvisational. Similar to the excerpt presented in figure 3.1, here biomedical understandings of HIV/AIDS are transposed to the context of choir rehearsals. In this case, though, the HIV-positive status of choir members is less implicit as group members laugh about the clumsy dancing of one of the group members.

It is early March 2008. I am video-recording a rehearsal for the very first time. The choir has been rehearsing for over an hour, running through songs with which they are already familiar. Amahle, Bongiwe, Celokuhle, and Zethu are present, as are male choir members Lethu, Ndumiso, Philani, Siphesihle, and Thulani. In the midst of a sticky Durban summer, it is hot in the garage. Everyone is sweating and needs to take a break to sit down and drink some water. As soon as the song ends, Bongiwe asks (the conversation is spoken in isiZulu, translated here), "Do you see that Lethu kicked me?" (Bongiwe has been kicked on her lower leg.)

Thulani starts to laugh in a high-pitched chuckle. Lethu is about ten years younger than the other choir members, and the most recent addition to the group. He has been recruited to sing bass, since Siphesihle and Philani have chosen to play the bass guitar and piano to be able to perform in a contemporary gospel style. The fact that Lethu is a novice is significant because it means that he has had less experience with the group choreography (discussed later in the chapter).

Lethu responds with incredulity, "Me?"

Bongiwe overlaps with Lethu's response, ready to continue her joke regardless of what Lethu says. She explains, "A person who comes close here will truly be infected again."

Thulani starts laughing again, this time in an even higher pitch.

"You were kicked by me?" Lethu asks, skeptical of Bongiwe's account.

"Don't you see that this is blood?" Bongiwe replies.

Thulani says (in English), "Seriously?"

Simultaneously, Bongiwe continues, "I have a problem," while Lethu questions her, "Where did I kick you?"

"By my shoe," Bongiwe laughs. Lethu joins in the laughter too.

Thulani closes the joking, exclaiming, "*Eish eish!*" (In this context, this is an isiZulu expression of disbelief.) "You will leave us as you are sitting down there, you."

In this exchange, there were two bits of implicit knowledge that shaped the collaborative unfolding of the joke. The first involved the fact that a semi-professional singer/dancer should be proficient enough not to step on other members of the group. As the youngest and least experienced member of the group, Lethu was singled out and teased for his mistake in stepping on Bongiwe's leg. The second involved biomedical models of HIV/AIDS. The joke relied on the knowledge that HIV/AIDS can be spread through the exchange of blood. Additionally, Bongiwe implicitly disclosed the HIV-positive status of group members when she used the isiZulu word *futhi* ("again"—a person who comes close here will truly be infected **again**). This implied that group members were already living with HIV. Through this collaborative joking exchange, Thembeka choir members reflected on their understandings of HIV/AIDS and fine-tuned shared ideals of an attitude to not take their status too seriously—to live positively.

While the previous example of joking about HIV was embodied in the sense that all speech is embodied, this example also involved an orientation toward bodies and bodily fluids. Choir members were exhausted from the exertion of rehearsal in the summer heat. They had been synchronizing voices and bodies (yet to be discussed) as they made music together. Bongiwe had gotten hurt, and was calling attention to a small laceration on her leg. There was thus an embodied element to the reflexive transposition of HIV into this rehearsal context also.

HUMOR IN EMBODIED CONFRONTATIONS WITH HEGEMONIC MASCULINITY

The following examples of joking focused not on HIV itself but on alternative understandings of masculinity that emerged in the context of group members' work in HIV support and activist organizations. In their activist roles, both men and women of the choir confronted ideologies of hypersexual masculinity that were significant in the South African AIDS epidemic. However, men in the choir tended to have a difficult time fully abandoning such dominant tropes. Here, "hegemonic masculinity" refers to ideas and embodied feelings about men and manhood (often held by both men and women) that contribute to patriarchy and male dominance—that is, to gendered inequities (Connell and Messerschmidt 2005; Speer 2001). Previous research theorizes how persons' engagement with new medical technologies and options may lead them to reexamine hegemonic masculinities and embody "emergent masculinities" as they opt in or opt out of biomedical treatment (Inhorn and Wentzell 2011; Rosenfeld and Faircloth 2006). In South Africa in 2008, hegemonic Zulu masculinity included ideologies of male hypersexuality. In line with idealized notions of a Zulu tradition of polygamy, heterosexual men were often expected to have multiple sexual partners (Hunter 2005; Meintjes 2004). These expectations, when enacted, contributed to the spread of HIV. Such ideals of hegemonic masculinity were sometimes critiqued when men took up roles in HIV support and activist organizations (Moolman 2013; Robins 2008). Similarly, choir members sometimes played with alternative conceptualizations of masculinity as they joked about HIV.

"As Any Other Boy"

It is October 2008. I have arranged to interview Philani. He is staying in Pietermaritzburg, where he now works for TB Leaders. Co-led by a choir member and an American doctor, TBL focuses on HIV and TB co-incidence, working with patients who are living with both HIV and TB (I discuss TBL further in chapter 4). I drive to Pietermaritzburg with Amahle and Elizabeth Falconi, who is an anthropologist in her own right and is visiting from the United States. We stop at the apartment where Philani is staying. I am expecting to do the interview there in the privacy of a separate room. Philani insists on going to a nearby mall to get some lunch.

When we sit down in a booth at the busy fast-food restaurant in the mall, it is clear that Philani expects to do the interview right then and there, with other customers and employees all around. The audience for Philani's interview thus includes Elizabeth and me (two white American anthropologists), Amahle, and the people that Philani imagined might hear the interview in the future (e.g., students, doctors, other academics). In addition, there are a number of potential overhearers—customers and employees at the fast-food restaurant. Analysis of the interview in this context can therefore reveal significant facets of Philani's social world, including what he was willing to say in a public space and how he shaped his stories for the various audiences at play.

I begin our interview by asking Philani how men's difficulties with HIV compare with women's difficulties with HIV. He suggests that men have more problems with HIV because they, unlike women, do not go to the doctor for prenatal visits. I then ask Philani to talk a little about how he grew up. About three and a half minutes into the interview, I am struggling to articulate my next question. I say, "Ahm, what was I going to ask? And, how did you—"

"Whether I had girlfriends by then?" Philani overlaps humorously, offering a potential next topic. I laugh.

"At one stage I had about twelve of them," he continues. "Because it was more like a game to us a long time ago, before all these things."

"Like *isoka*?" I ask. *Isoka* is an isiZulu word that is often translated as "boy-friend." However, the term implies that a man has more than one girlfriend. Another translation might be "player-boyfriend." The corresponding word for a woman with multiple boyfriends is a slur.

"Yeah," Philani agrees. "It was, there was nothing wrong with . . . having many girlfriends and having all these things up until this AIDS thing came and people then started to . . . to get educated and know some of the things, but as any other boy I had more than one or two. But then that's why, in the first question asked, it was a little bit difficult but I did know that. I knew my ways, so there should be consequences along those ways. So that's why it wasn't that difficult for me."

Here, Philani relied on stereotypes of hegemonic masculinity to address the delicate topic of how he became infected with HIV and what his sexual life was like prior to his infection even as he critiqued these stereotypes. He balanced the two by telling a turning-point narrative (see Capps and Ochs 1995). In some ways, this mirrored the stories told by Bongiwe and Amahle in which becoming a member of the choir and support group provided the basis for a turning point. Philani told a story in which he was depicted as normal, like other boys, and as a normal boy he made a game of trying to have as many partners as possible. He even suggested that there was nothing wrong with this practice before the AIDS pandemic descended upon South Africa. The turning point of this story came when AIDS forced people "to get educated." Given the continuing prevalence of sex with multiple partners and sex without condoms in South Africa, this turning point may have been less a statement of fact than a way for Philani to incorporate his current social role of an AIDS activist/educator into his story. The interview was, after all, being recorded for future audiences, and Amahle (a shrewd and discerning judge of choir members' activist tendencies) was also sitting right next to Philani. Working to reconcile this turning-point narrative with his earlier response that men had a more difficult time with HIV than women, Philani oscillated between saying that he knew the error of his ways but also that "it was a little bit difficult." Philani's post–support group shift in his understanding of Zulu masculinity matches the findings of other anthropological research about gender and HIV/AIDS. That scholarship suggests that engagement with nonprofits and other groups that promote the moral/ethical framework of rights and responsibilities may lead South Africans to critically rethink dominant sexual politics (Robins 2008: ch. 7). Novel configurations of masculinity or confrontations with hegemonic masculinity may also emerge as individuals and groups engage with newly available technologies and treatments (Inhorn and Wentzell 2011).

"And Then He Went for a Checkup"

Comparing Philani's story about HIV infection to others I heard during fieldwork, I found that both men and women sometimes relied on stereotypes associated with hegemonic masculinity to tell the most awkward or embarrassing parts of their stories about HIV. Philani was apologetic but reasoned that this was just the way things were in South Africa before HIV/AIDS. Often, women were not so sympathetic. The next example of joking comes from a group interview conducted by Amahle with some of her women neighbors who were HIV positive. Amahle was the only person to which some of these women had initially disclosed their HIV status. This interview was conducted in isiZulu with women who were not choir members, providing a window into isiZulu patterns of discourse about HIV that were a degree more distant from the activist projects and institutional frameworks of choir members.

It is September 2008. Amahle and I meet with three of her neighbors in the living room of her home in the township. Amahle and I sit with the three women, Nombuso, Thabile, and Zandile, on beige fabric couches that are pushed up against three of the walls of the room. A large set of cabinets with curios and an entertainment system occupy the fourth wall. The curtains are drawn on windows that face the front of the house. I sit in silence while Amahle conducts the interview. I have not worked with Amahle to develop a clear set of questions or a sense of how to not "lead the witness," so to speak, by implying certain answers in the questions. Without this guidance or previous interviewer experience, many of her questions are value laden and direct her interviewees in particular ways. One of the first questions that Amahle poses to her three neighbors is, "Your partner knows about your HIV status?" The preferred response to Amahle is clearly "yes," implying that the interviewee has been a responsible person and informed her partner of her HIV-positive diagnosis. This is indicative of Amahle's stance on activism and HIV disclosure. Commentary on the gendered division of responses to HIV infection ensues after she asks this question.

In response to Amahle's question (presented in figure 3.2), Zandile uses wry humor to indicate her evaluation of her partner's response to her HIV-positive diagnosis. She indicates to the others that they should interpret her story as humorous when she laughs (in line 05) after saying that she was "compelled" (*ngabe*) to go straight to him. Then she repeats, "I was compelled to give it [the result] to him." In lines 05 and 06, Zandile voices her partner's response, changing her intonational pattern to produce an imitation of a man stuttering through an attempt to explain her recent sickness without talking about HIV. Zandile indicates that her partner dismissed her sickness as diarrhea. She uses scatological humor and refers to diarrhea, a common side effect of opportunistic infections that impact people living with HIV. Amahle picks up on the humor and adds onomatopoeia of the in-progress humor and speech play, using the word *bupepepe* to refer to the diarrhea (the "peh peh peh" at the end of the word sounds like liquid dropping into a toilet). Zandile ends her account by explaining, "and then he went for a checkup." This statement implies the inevitability of her partner's infection despite his denial. She did not have to say that he was found to be HIV positive. It is expected.

In this example, the women's joking about a man's bumbling response (and his assertion that his partner's HIV infection was just diarrhea) relied on the implicit notion that (South African) men lacked responsibility and practiced widespread infidelity. This was, in essence, the same stereotype associated with hegemonic masculinity that Philani relied upon when talking about his own HIV infection. But where Philani accepted infidelity and lack of responsibility as a value-neutral part of his pre-HIV masculine persona (boys will be boys), in the women had a strong negative evaluation of that sort of persona, as is evident in figure 3.2.

This *Shima* Thing of Yours

In the context of HIV/AIDS, then, attitudes about masculinity and promiscuity often became associated with stances on HIV infection and blame. Recognizing this association, choir members sometimes played with hegemonic Zulu masculinity in the course of rehearsals. The following example of joking occurred just after the joking discussed in figure 3.1. While I recount the conversation here in English translation, it was spoken in isiZulu.

Remember that Bongiwe has been sweeping the floor in preparation for choir rehearsal and joking with Ndumiso about TB. As Bongiwe continues

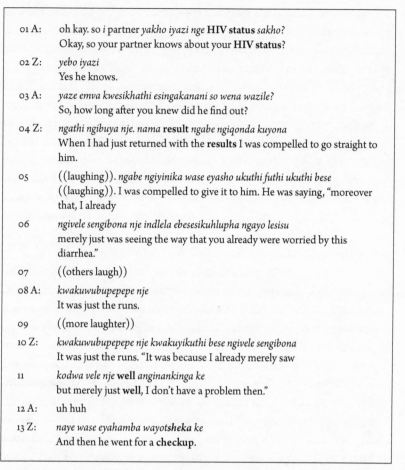

01 A: oh kay. so *i* partner *yakho iyazi nge* **HIV status** *sakho?*
       Okay, so your partner knows about your **HIV status**?

02 Z: *yebo iyazi*
       Yes he knows.

03 A: *yaze emva kwesikhathi esingakanani so wena wazile?*
       So, how long after you knew did he find out?

04 Z: *ngathi ngibuya nje. nama* **result** *ngabe ngiqonda kuyona*
       When I had just returned with the **results** I was compelled to go straight to him.

05   ((laughing)). *ngabe ngiyinika wase eyasho ukuthi futhi ukuthi bese*
       ((laughing)). I was compelled to give it to him. He was saying, "moreover that, I already

06   *ngivele sengibona nje indlela ebesesikuhlupha ngayo lesisu*
       merely just was seeing the way that you already were worried by this diarrhea."

07   ((others laugh))

08 A: *kwakuwubupepepe nje*
       It was just the runs.

09   ((more laughter))

10 Z: *kwakuwubupepepe nje kwakuyikuthi bese ngivele sengibona*
       It was just the runs. "It was because I already merely saw

11   *kodwa vele nje* **well** *anginankinga ke*
       but merely just **well**, I don't have a problem then."

12 A: uh huh

13 Z: *naye wase eyahamba wayotsheka ke*
       And then he went for a **checkup**.

FIGURE 3.2. Transcript: It Was Merely the Runs (interview/conversation 9-11-2008, 2 min 52 sec). Participants (all female): A = Amahle, N = Nombuso, T = Thabile, Z = Zandile, English code-mixing indicated in bold.

to sweep the floor of the garage/choir rehearsal space, she sweeps near Philani. He reacts, asking (in isiZulu), "Why don't you say move if you are coming near me?"

Bongiwe replies, "It's because of this *shima* thing of yours, that you are a *shima*, and then you say it was caused by me." *Shima* is derived from the isiZulu term *isishimane*, which refers to an adult that has no romantic partners, and more specifically a person who is unable to attract a partner. In Zulu understandings of health and illness, as previously mentioned, sweeping dust toward a person may cause not only physical but also psychological illness, so that a person might have a problem, such as finding a partner. Drawing from this idea again as she sweeps, Bongiwe both playfully insults Philani and implies that now Philani would have an excuse for why he is a *shima*.

Egged on by this playful insult to his sexuality and masculinity, Philani insists, "Me, I'm the leader of the *soka* here. If *sokas* are being talked about in this room." Bongiwe and Philani both laugh. Remember that the term *soka* refers to a man who has multiple partners and values a man's ability to have more than one girlfriend. It is also the default term for "boyfriend." In contrast, the default term for "girlfriend," *intombi*, refers to a girl with only one boyfriend, and remember that the term for a woman with multiple boyfriends is considerably more negative in tone. These indexical values of the words for "boyfriend" and "girlfriend" provide clues to how hypersexuality and hegemonic masculinity are linked in this context.

Philani and Bongiwe continue in this vein, going back and forth, with Philani insisting that he is a *soka*. He explains that he was born being a *soka*, that he leads the *sokas* but is subtle and quiet about his sexual exploits. Meanwhile, Bongiwe playfully ignores him and continues to talk about his *shima* problem.

Then Bongiwe shifts her conversational footing (Goffman 1974), stating, "The female body part, it is a curse." She turns to talk again to Ndumiso, explaining, "because we have a bad reputation, Ndumiso, as you see us."

Dumisile, a choir member who is a woman, joins the conversation at this point, asking, "It's like, if you talk about the female private part, it is a curse, but for a male person the private part is not a curse. What's the deal?" Dumisile and Ndumiso laugh together. "What's the deal, just all women have a curse?"

Ndumiso replies, "It's because the man's parts are important." This statement closes the playful encounter. At this point, a side conversation that I have been having with Philani takes center stage, and the other choir members' talk about gender and sexuality stops.

This exchange took place with the background knowledge that men and women both understood heterosexual males to be promiscuous but that men and women differentially valued or devalued that promiscuity, as the terms *isishimane*, *isoka*, and *intombi* demonstrate. When I spoke with men, even those who were in monogamous relationships and those who worked as HIV activists, they tended to display similar elements of hegemonic masculinity. Women, on the other hand, often critiqued men's tendency to have multiple romantic partners, but still accepted it as normal if undesirable. This idealization and valuing of male promiscuity was particularly problematic in the context of the HIV epidemic, where it could lead to the further spread of HIV infection. The ABCs of HIV prevention included Abstain, Be faithful, and Condomize. Male promiscuity was clearly not in line with the "B" of the ABCs.

In conversation about *shimas* and *sokas*, group members played with ideas about masculinity that were alternative to hegemonic ideals. In the context of choir rehearsal, Ndumiso and Philani were able to joke with female choir members Bongiwe and Dumisile about stereotypical notions of masculine sexual prowess and thereby to critique corresponding negative attitudes toward female sexuality (exploring the term that refers to a woman's private parts). Alternative notions of heterosexual masculinity emerged out of the embodied reflexive interplay between group members in the choir rehearsal space before choir rehearsal began. Though Ndumiso's comment ended the joking with a (humorous) reinforcement of hegemonic masculinity ("the man's parts are important"), group members had the opportunity to embody, through linguistic performance, distinct understandings of masculinity and femininity that confronted the hegemony of valuing male promiscuity—distinct understandings that were an important part of HIV activism. As in the other examples of joking about HIV, collaborative, improvisational exchange yielded an embodied reflexive instantiation of biosociality, this time inflected with more critical and explicit reflection on gender stereotypes and their applicability in contexts of HIV support and activism.

More generally, group members' joking about HIV was an embodied, reflexive genre of performance that was specific to the choir community. This was a community of people who shared ways of speaking about HIV—a bio-speech community that cohered in part through a shared biomedical characteristic (a biosocial group). In the context of pervasive stigma, the embodied reflexivity of linguistic and musical performance helped this biosocial group to cohere. Reflexivity allowed group members to point toward HIV without discussing it outright. Choir members thereby constructed and maintained a community that was significantly oriented toward their experiences with HIV. I refer to this group as a bio-speech community not only to indicate the power of biomedicine in the creation and maintenance of this speech community but also to showcase how the specific properties of linguistic performance, including improvisational collaboration, an intermediate level of reflexivity, shaped the production of biosociality.

EMBODIMENT OF SUPPORT THROUGH SONG

Even more so than joking about HIV, singing about HIV provided a context for embodying biosociality as group members became immersed in the shared temporal flow of making music together. In response to stigma, support was (re)constituted when choir members made music together, their bodies—including their voices—moving in synchrony with one another. A common feature of the human capacity for musicality is immersion in a shared temporal flow. It is true that people have to attend to timing in all conversation (this is why a lag in a video call or phone call can be so disorienting); and it is also true that timing conventions are, to a certain extent, cultural (for instance, in the United States, northerners tend to overlap with one another in conversation or leave less of a gap between speakers than southerners and westerners). Still, making music together requires people to coordinate in a more intensive, self-aware manner, such that musicians can sing or play instruments *at the same time* rather than talking one at a time (Clayton et al. 2004; Schutz 1964). The coordination of timing is not only temporal but also spatial insofar as it is dependent upon the use of multiple semiotic resources—glances, foot tapping, head nods, and other bodily movements of co-performers. Each act of making music together is a symphony of multiple semiotic modalities.

Keeping a steady rhythmic beat shared among multiple participants is by no means a simple task. In different musical traditions, performers have developed distinct methods for doing so. For instance, the employment of a specialized participant—a conductor—who displays and to a certain extent controls the beat with a large number of other participants is a notable feature of Euro-classical orchestras. Jazz musicians often use the concept of "listening to one another" to conceptualize collaborative efforts at maintaining a steady rhythmic beat and coordinating actions. In the choir, stepping and swaying together was a way to keep time together. Even before they began to sing, vocalists of the choir would begin to step back and forth together in time with the music, swaying left and right. These footsteps and swaying were a way of keeping time together, similar to foot tapping in an orchestra or the regular steps in a marching band. Group members' regular pattern of stepping and swaying also produced an aesthetically valued choreography. This synchronized swaying and stepping was something that could be understood, appreciated, and enacted by any human, but the distinct meaning associated with swaying, stepping, and singing together as an embodiment of support was rooted in choir members' shared knowledge of each other's HIV-positive status. Here, I describe the moment-to-moment construction of embodied synchrony and explore how the cultural meaning of support and reflexive commentary about HIV were laminated onto this embodied synchrony.

Moving Together

It is May 2008. At choir rehearsal, group members are practicing a new song written by Siphesihle. The song is about stigma—about hearing people joking about HIV in negative ways, spreading medical misinformation about the virus, and avoiding talk about the illness altogether. Ndumiso is playing a steady four-beat pattern on the drums, with Siphesihle and Philani riffing on a classic southern African harmonic resolution on piano and bass.[1] I quickly turn my camera toward the floor to capture the vocalists' foot movements. Group members' footsteps form a pattern. On beat one group members move their right foot to their right (gray in figure 3.3); on beat two (unshaded, white in the figure) their left foot moves inward toward their right foot; on beat three (checkered) their left foot moves back to their left; and on beat four (speckled) their right foot moves inward toward their right foot. Generally, this foot movement pattern is employed whenever the choir is singing a song in which the rhythmic cycle is four beats.

This footstep pattern leads the vocalists to sway back and forth in synchrony with one another. Figure 3.4 represents this swaying movement. Here (taken from a different choir rehearsal), group members are represented by outlines of their bodies within the frame of the stationary video camera. Again, the shading inside these outlines corresponds to beats one through four. The three choir members on the left of the video frame move in synchrony with each other and the music, swaying/stepping first to their right, back to center, and then to their left. The choir member on the far right in

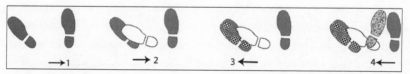

FIGURE 3.3. Stepping Together.

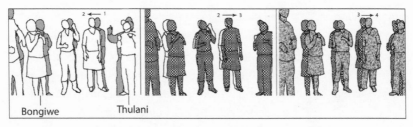

Bongiwe   Thulani

FIGURE 3.4. Swaying While Singing (5-17-2008, Tape 2, 19 min 9 sec).

each of the three diagrams, Thulani, is directing the vocalists and not sway-ing/stepping in exact synchrony with the other three group members.

Figure 3.5 combines the images of figure 3.4 to show choir members' body movement over the four beats (repeated) in the song. The absence of gray silhouettes in this synthesized figure (except Thulani's on the far right) dem-onstrates how body positioning on beat three is almost identical to body positioning on beat one as group members sway back and forth.

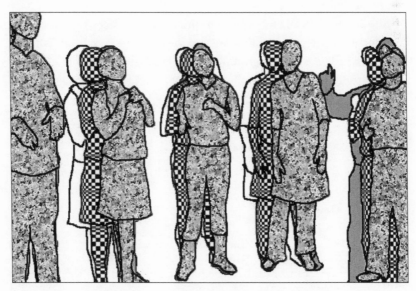

FIGURE 3.5. Body Positioning, Beats One through Four.

Finding Harmony

Harmonizing involves multiple participants' vocal cords being modulated to oscillate at complementary speeds, so harmonizing may also be understood as part of keeping time together: "bodies and brains synchronize gestures, muscle actions, breathing, and brain waves while enveloped in music" (Becker 2004: 135). These processes are clearest in instances where coordination is disrupted—when things go wrong or expectations are breached—and performers make efforts to re-establish coordination. Sometimes, as in the following example, choir members' efforts to re-establish embodied synchrony and coordinate rhythm and harmony resulted in embodied enactments of support.

It is May 17, 2008. At choir rehearsal, vocalists are swaying back and forth in time to the music. They are practicing the same song about HIV stigma described above. They begin to repeat sung lyrical phrases as they work on their harmonies together. In the midst of this musical action, Bongiwe opens her eyes wide and shakes her head back and forth to indicate no. She also stops singing while the others continue. When the other vocalists see Bongiwe's frustrated expression, they step closer to be able to hear one another. After a few more seconds of careful listening and adjusting, they resolve their harmonic difficulties.

The vocalists do all of this in time with the music, stepping toward one another at precisely the right moment in the four-beat pattern of footsteps described earlier. After Bongiwe shakes her head and widens her eyes, displaying trouble finding the tone she is supposed to be singing, Thulani

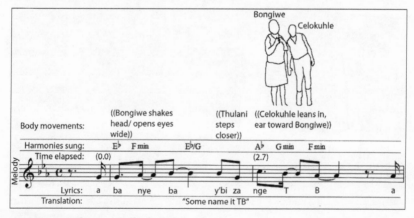

FIGURE 3.6. Indicating Difficulty While Singing.

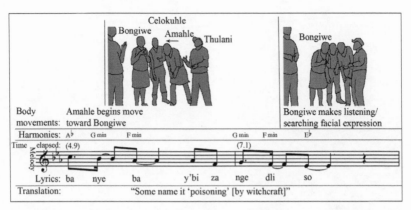

Body movements:	Amahle begins move toward Bongiwe			Bongiwe makes listening/ searching facial expression	

Harmonies:	A♭	G min	F min	G min	F min	E♭

Time elapsed:	(4.9)			(7.1)		

Lyrics:	ba	nye	ba	y'bi	za	nge	dli	so

Translation:	"Some name it 'poisoning' [by witchcraft]"

FIGURE 3.7. Troubleshooting While Singing.

responds by stepping closer to her. Celokuhle then leans in toward Bongiwe in spatial synchrony. Celokuhle orients her ear rather than her eyes toward Bongiwe's face (as shown in the tracing in figure 3.6), directing her attention to the harmonies being sung.[2]

After this, Amahle also steps close in synchrony with the group's choreography, and these choir members then huddle together as they sing (see figure 3.7). Thulani yells to get the group to repeat these lyrics a third time to finish fixing the harmonic problem. The next and final cycle is notable. Bongiwe stands up straight, showing the others that her trouble finding her part has been resolved, but Celokuhle and Amahle do not move from their huddled body positioning. Instead, Celokuhle wraps her left arm around Amahle's back, holding her in position, and smiles as they sing together (figure 3.8).

In this moment of rehearsal, musical trouble led to physical proximity as group members paid close attention to one another's vocal actions (the precise tuning of vocal cord vibrations). This in turn became an occasion to display a social relationship of closeness and affinity through the physical support of each other's bodies in synchrony with the movement of other choir members. As mentioned, choir members regularly commented to me that no matter what was going on in their lives, they always had this once-a-week pause in their daily lives where they could lose themselves in song. Part of the choir's enjoyment came from the physical activity, similar to how one might find relief and relaxation in a long run or a trip to the gym. Part of their enjoyment came from the feeling of support that they got from engaging in this embodied activity together. No one had to talk about

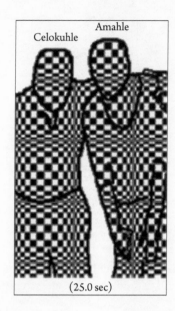

FIGURE 3.8. Support While Singing.

HIV—they had already done that over the years, first in support group meetings with counselors and doctors at Durban Hospital HIV clinic and later in the interstices of choir rehearsals—but one could feel free to do so, knowing that everyone at the rehearsal was living with HIV. And finally, as they told me, part of their enjoyment came from making music, including the embodied synchronicity demonstrated in the foregoing analysis. Through this togetherness and embodied engagement, choir members promoted a sense of support.

Lyrical Transpositions

As with joking about HIV, singing about HIV was not only embodied but also reflexive. Much of the music that the choir practiced was broadly classified as Zulu gospel music. This included popular gospel songs with lyrics such as, "*ncwele ncwele somandla*" ("holy, holy Almighty") and songs written by choir members with lines such as, "we are praying to the lion of Judah, *saphel' isizwe*" ("we are praying to Jesus, the nation is finished"). Group members understood Christianity (of many varieties, e.g., Episcopal, Catholic, Pentecostal, Evangelical) to be the default among them (Christianity, faith, and understandings of HIV/AIDS are discussed in chapter 5). Additionally, some songs written by choir members lamented the HIV epidemic in general, in

01	*Into enjani lena, into enjani lena* The thing that is like what, the thing that is like what
02	*Okukhulunywa ngayo* That is talked about [repeated 2×]
03	*Abanye bahlekisa ngayo* Some are laughing about it
04	*bayibiza ngeqhoks* ((*iqhoks* = "high heel")) They are calling it *iqhoks* ((some are teasing about it))
05	*Bayibiza ngamagama amathathu* They are calling it "a three letter word" ((HIV)) [repeated 2×]
06	*Abanye bayibiza nge*-TB Some are calling it TB
07	*Abanye bayibiza ngedliso* Some are calling it poisoning ((by witchcraft)) [repeated 2×]
08	*Waze wangiyala, wangiyala wengculazi* How you are bothering me, You, AIDS, are bothering me
09	*Ngibengisathe ngibathe kukhulunywa ngami* Whatever I do, they are talking about me [repeated 2×]

FIGURE 3.9. Transcript: The Thing That Is Talked About.

ways that were broadly similar to popular songs that were well-known among South Africans; and one choir song focused on the group's experiences with international aid.

In particular, the lyrics in the song displayed in figures 3.6 to 3.8 were remarkable in their metalinguistic commentary on stigmatizing reference to HIV. These lyrics critiqued dominant discourses in which people used "TB" and "*idliso*" (witchcraft) to avoid directly referring to HIV. The lyrics are reproduced in full in figure 3.9, with English translations.

The first line of the song refers indirectly to HIV. This immediately invokes stigmatization and avoidance of direct discussion of HIV (discussed in chapter 6). HIV is indexed as "the thing that is like what, that is talked about." In line 02, the verb *ukukhuluma* ("to talk") takes a relative prefix ("that"), which links it to the previous line, and a passive suffix:[3]

Oku-	khulu-	nywa	ngayo
Rel.n15	talk	PAS	about

"That is talked about"

The first verse (lines 01–02) is thus notable for its absence of a grammatical agent. In verses two and three, the lack of an agent is replaced by the general pronoun *abanye* ("some"/"somebody"). This indefinite pronoun is the subject and semantic agent that jokes about HIV and names HIV using terms of avoidance such as *iqhoks* (the sound of high-heeled shoes), *amagama amathathu* ("a three letter word"), TB, and *idliso* (poisoning by witchcraft). I discuss these terms and their indexical valences in depth in chapters 5 and 6. Here, I note that the identification of joking about HIV and reference to HIV as TB as stigmatized forms of reference suggests that the ways that choir members joked about HIV and TB were creative transformations of stigma. These terms were linked to the biomedical and traditional Zulu understandings of HIV in the examples of joking about HIV discussed earlier. Describing the virus as either TB or witchcraft not only yielded aversion but also led people to avoid frank discussion about the illness, its biomedical causes, prevention techniques, and treatment. The indirect metalinguistic reflexivity of the song lyrics (e.g., "some" call it TB) was diffused across multiple participants who were singing together and simultaneously embodying support through vocal harmonization and rhythmic entrainment. Similar to the indirection and diffusion of responsibility evident in collaborative joking, this form of distributed, highly embodied reflexivity may have functioned to help choir members face stigma by allowing the group to voice commentary on a stigmatized topic while distancing individual group members from responsibility for that commentary.

BIO-SPEECH COMMUNITIES: BIOSOCIALITY IN AND THROUGH LANGUAGE

The Thembeka choir was able to cohere as a support group throughout the 2000s when others living with HIV were struggling. Group members tended to avoid many of the most extreme psychological impacts of stigma and HIV diagnosis, where others near to them, including siblings and spouses, succumbed to depression and, in one case, suicide. One question I and others asked was why this was the case. Clearly, music played a role. Rather than simply stating the truism that music and humor heal, though, the foregoing examination of embodied reflexivity in choir member encounters provides a more precise and helpful answer. The organization of embodied reflexivity in performance provided a mix of interpersonal engagement and communicative distance that helped group members to face stigma and thereby be able to communicate about HIV with one another.

In terms of the classic speech community model—frequent interaction, shared verbal repertoire, and shared norms of language use (or language ideologies)—in this chapter I have focused primarily on frequent interactions (weekly choir rehearsals) and shared verbal repertoire. In particular, I have examined how the choir's verbal repertoire was centered around ways of speaking that enacted biosociality by engaging directly with biomedical discourses. Joking and singing were two genres that formed key parts of the group's verbal repertoire. These genres provided ways for choir members to transpose HIV into choir rehearsals. The genres allowed group members to reflect upon traditional Zulu and biomedical models of health and illness, as well as patterns of stigmatization and AIDS activism, in a collective forum where understandings were displayed not usually through overt narrative discussion but rather through the temporal unfolding of communicative encounters. While there was patterned variation between men and women, the group as a whole tended to affiliate with the perspectives associated with relatively powerful global health discourses and they displayed that affiliation through the transposition of biomedical models of HIV/AIDS and TB into isiZulu encounters. At the same time, they still lived in home communities where the threat of stigma was ever-present. Through spoken and sung performance, the choir was able to position itself ideologically as linked to both global health and home communities.

Collaborative joking about HIV diffused responsibility for talk about the virus across multiple conversational participants. Furthermore, the fact that the "secondary text" of jokes usually remained implicit but recognized made it possible to orient to shared understandings of HIV without articulating those understandings outright. As choir members responded meaningfully to talk about TB, dust, and Zulu masculinity, they demonstrated their familiarity with a constellation of concepts associated with traditional Zulu understandings of illness while simultaneously displaying a critical stance (rooted in familiarity with biomedicine) toward those understandings. These attitudes and stances were entextualized in song lyrics that were embodied as group members vocalized in harmony with one another. Embodied reflexivity was central to the creation and maintenance of a shared verbal repertoire that included ways of transposing HIV by joking about and singing about the virus. In other words, embodied reflexivity yielded biosociality amid stigma. This shared verbal repertoire contributed to the maintenance of a bio-speech community oriented toward HIV support and AIDS activism.

4 · THE POWER OF GLOBAL HEALTH AUDIENCES

It is July 2008. I wake up and check my email. I read a note from Laura, an American doctor who has lived in South Africa for quite some time. Laura has dedicated her life to HIV treatment and prevention. She previously worked with the Durban Hospital clinic and met choir members there. She started out with little funding, using her personal research funding—likely from the prestigious Ivy League university with which she was associated— to pay for staff. Now, Laura and choir member Fanele lead a small, innovative nonprofit organization based in Pietermaritzburg, TB Leaders (TBL). TBL utilizes patient-activists such as Fanele as expert transposers of the bio-medical models of HIV/AIDS and TB. These TBL employees translate between isiZulu and English and interpret the intersection between Zulu tra-ditional models and biomedical models of illness as they work with HIV/ TB patients. Recently, two other choir members, Philani and Zethu, have begun working as counselors for TBL. To do so, they first were required to complete intensive training to pass a crash course on biomedical models of HIV and TB.

In her email, Laura questions me about my videography skills and asks if I can come to Pietermaritzburg to meet with her. With my somewhat rudi-mentary MiniDV video camera and Mac laptop, I had made a few DVDs for choir members and other support group members. One DVD had some songs from choir rehearsal on it, one had a video from a choir member's birth-day on it, and one featured the wedding of two former choir members.

Laura was planning a promotional video for TBL, and Philani mentioned my DVD projects to her. Excited to learn more about TBL and expand my research, I write back that I am available all day. Laura promptly replies, asking me to come in at 11 A.M.

After I make the one-hour drive to Pietermaritzburg and find my way to the TBL offices, I meet Laura for the first time. She strikes me as a no-nonsense, work-driven person. I pull out my laptop and start to show her the DVDs I have made for choir members. Soon after I begin, Laura stops me, politely but in no uncertain terms informing me that she needs a "professional quality" video. She mentions that most professionally edited videos have at least three different tracks running simultaneously (e.g., video, soundtrack, and voice-over). My videos feature almost no audio-editing. Laura explains that this video will be going to potential donors in the United States—people who want to see a polished product. I am a little puzzled by this: if an organization can afford a highly edited, professional video, I would think that it means the organization does not need donations as much as a group that cannot afford such a production.

Despite her critique of my videos, or maybe because of it, Laura kindly invites me to observe interviews with patients that have benefited from TBL's work, interviews that will be recorded and edited to create the TBL promotional video. The next day, I get back in the car and drive to a medical facility near Pinetown (a town outside of Durban) to watch the interviews. The interviews are held in the chapel of the medical facility, perhaps for sound and lighting and perhaps to link the charitable contributions with faith-based aid. Laura sits and asks the patients leading questions. The professional camera operator films over her shoulder, so that the interviewee is almost looking at the camera. The interviewees repeat Laura's questions before answering them, so that only the aid recipients' voices will be heard in the edited video. Interviewees talk about how good it feels to be alive, referring to donors as angels and the best people in the world or universe. Laura and her interviewees know what I do not: that aid givers want production value. They want to be wooed and to know they are contributing to something that is demonstrably successful.

This brief vignette is just one instance of a broader pattern, wherein individuals, groups, and institutions associated with global health crafted their presentations of self—both through media and in face-to-face encounters—in order to be attractive to powerful global health audiences. It demonstrates a stark global health hierarchy in which certain groups (primarily those of the global North) acted as audiences who implicitly shaped global health discourses because they had the power, wealth, and connections to support health interventions. Here, I examine how Thembeka choir members' stories and musical performances were shaped by these audiences, discussing what happened in encounters with powerful global health professionals. I discuss how inequity impacted patient-activists' engagement with global health professional and donor audiences, especially examining the process of audience-design. Linking scholarship on the language ideological construction of the "global" in global health (Brada 2011); research on the dynamics of uneven transnational circulation of people, medicine, discourses, and money associated with global health (e.g., Briggs 2011; Hörbst and Gerrits 2016; Nguyen 2010); and analysis of audience design and the power of the listening subject (e.g., Bell and Gibson 2011; Duranti and Brenneis 1986; Inoue 2003), this chapter examines how global health groups functioned as imagined and actual audiences that shaped the contours of global health discourses.

THE ANTHROPOLOGY OF AUDIENCES AND LISTENERS

Anthropological scholarship on audiences, addressees, and listeners emphasizes the significant role played by interlocutors even when they are not speaking. Listening is not merely an act of aural reception. Rather, culture and power shape who counts as a relevant or significant addressee, how speakers change or do not change their talk in response to these significant addressees, and how listeners display their aural attention (Duranti and Brenneis 1986; Inoue 2003; Marsilli-Vargas 2014). As Alessandro Duranti (1986) writes, "Interpretation is not conceived as the speaker's privilege. On the contrary, it is based on the ability (and power) that others may have to invoke certain conventions, to establish links between different acts and different social personae" (241). Though an analysis of power and hierarchy is evident in this analysis of listening, it was not until more recently that scholarship began to focus on issues of audience authority and ideology, discussing the significance of powerful listeners' evaluations in the constitution of culturally specific subjectivities (e.g., Inoue 2003). Here, the power of auditory attention is intertwined with the hegemony of the "gaze" of authority. This is a gaze that shapes the double-consciousness of marginalized individuals as they must constantly be oriented both toward other members of the marginalized group and toward the evaluative frameworks imposed by dominant groups (Du Bois 2008 [1903]; Gilroy 1993; Piot 2001). In South Africa as in other parts of the world, the authoritative gaze of white individuals has been described as impacting marginalized persons' actions and cultural standpoints in just these sorts of ways (Hansen 2012). In this chapter, I analyze (primarily white) global health audiences as listeners whose social authority and access to resources had similar impacts on marginalized black South African patient-activists living with HIV.

Within this orientation to global health audiences, I focus especially on these processes in contexts of performance. As mentioned in previous chapters, research distinguishes between two kinds of performance: everyday and staged (Bell and Gibson 2011). In staged performance, linguistic patterns, location, or other aspects of context invoke a performer/audience dichotomy in which a performer "holds the floor" while (often implicitly) directing audience attention toward the aesthetics of speech or song (Bauman 1975). In everyday performance, there is less of a dichotomy between performers and audiences. Still, speakers generally frame talk in ways that direct addressees' attention toward an evaluation of the aesthetics of talk (Shuck 2004). Choral singing is a clear example of staged performance, where the social activity is oriented toward performance itself. Joking in conversation (e.g., the joking about HIV described in the previous chapter) is an example of everyday performance. While joking about HIV was primarily oriented toward other choir members as an audience, singing about HIV was primarily oriented toward and sensitive to the potential evaluation of global health audiences.

Responsiveness to evaluation, where performers craft the aesthetics of communication to appeal to particular imagined and actual audiences, has been labeled "audience design" (Bell 1984, 2011). In this chapter, I link the concept of audience design with the idea of "global health" as an ideological invention that often functions to reinforce existing hierarchies (Benton 2015; Brada 2011). My analysis of Thembeka choir members' performances for global health audiences provides insight into the ways that patient-activists were subtly, and perhaps unintentionally, localized and marginalized from global health intervention efforts. This analysis also demonstrates how the verbal repertoire of the choir (as a bio-speech community) was shaped by the power dynamics embedded in performer-audience encounters.

SOUTH AFRICAN DOCTORS AS A NONRESPONSIVE AUDIENCE

Providing evidence of how audiences and listeners shape encounters can be difficult, because in many cases speakers and performers may implicitly orient toward the power of audiences (more to come on this). However, in a few instances I was able not only to observe how global health audiences interacted with the Thembeka choir but also to discuss these encounters with choir members after the fact. One of the most notable encounters in this regard was a performance in which Durban Hospital staff misnamed the choir, referring to them by the name the choir had used when they had previously been associated with the hospital. When the group officially parted ways with the hospital they changed the choir's name. Across cultural contexts, how people refer to persons, places, and other entities is a significant aspect of the culturally specific organization of social groups (Basso 1988; Bucholtz 2016; Rymes 1996). In South Africa, Zulu personal names were often evocative of the social world into which a child was born (Suzman 1994). Family names (i.e., last names) held special value in Zulu tradition, forming the basis for an elaborate system of praise-name poetics that could be invoked at important ceremonies and celebrations (Koopman 2002). Most choir members, like many Zulu South Africans, had both an isiZulu name and an English or "church" name. In the early to mid-2000s, some individuals preferred to be called by their English names (De Klerk and Lagonikos 2004). Still, this tradition of having two names was rooted in the historical imposition of Christianity, the white South African insistence on the dominance of English and Afrikaans, and a tendency for at least some white South Africans to avoid learning more isiZulu than was necessary to issue commands (Adendorff 2002). In such a context, I interpret the inability or unwillingness of hospital staff to correctly address the Thembeka choir as a product of the powerful aural "gaze" of authority. In this case, global health professionals had the power to *not* listen—to ignore what choir members heard as a significant linguistic distinction that was supposed to have indexed an important shift in their relationship with Durban Hospital.

Misnaming While Introducing the Thembeka Choir

As mentioned, little of the Thembeka choir's name change conflict was evident during most of my time in South Africa. Other than my initial difficulty in contacting the choir, the first indication I saw of the conflict occurred late in my fieldwork when the choir was hired to perform at a medical conference organized by Durban Hospital that focused on HIV. I went with the choir to the performance and videotaped the occasion.

It is early October 2008. The hotel where the conference is being held is near the beautiful Durban beachfront, in a high-rise tower similar to others in the area. Choir members struggle to find the location and to arrive in time to prepare as a result of the difficulties of using public transportation. I help some individuals get to the performance on time, driving back and forth to the central downtown taxi rank to shuttle choir members to the hotel. Not all of the choir is able to be here—three of the men and four of the women are present. At the hotel, group members go into the bathrooms to change into their performance outfits.

The conference includes several booths where groups presenting new HIV medical treatments and studies have set up information tables, and in the lobby there is a cornucopia of coffee and muffins. Choir members are familiar with this sort of setup, and have performed at such events many times before, as evident in a question Philani asks me: "Steve, why are all these conferences exactly the same? Same food, same coffee, same everything."

The choir is warming up in the foyer, when a white South African woman walks by on her way to the bathroom. "Hello!" she says with a smile. Philani turns, waves, and says "hello" in return. The group is clearly focused on working out their respective parts for the performance.

Inattentive with respect to the group's intent focus on preparing for their performance, the woman continues, "This is very fun. Bring back old memories" (without conjugating the verb "bring"). Choir members laugh appreciatively. Without knowing her or her communicative patterns, it is impossible to extrapolate any definitive meaning behind the lack of a grammatical subject and lack of verbal conjugation in her interjection ("bring back" rather than "it brings back"). However, these patterns are consistent with the sorts of linguistic simplification that people sometimes enact when they think that they are speaking to nonproficient speakers of English. The woman continues on her way.

Soon after, the choir is called into the main conference room. The choir stands at the back of the room, waiting and talking to one of the doctors from the hospital. There are very few black South Africans in the room other than the choir members. Most conference attendees are white or Indian South Africans. Rows of tables stretch out in front of the group, a bottle of water and a conference folder carefully placed in front of each seat. Small clusters of scholars and doctors are spread throughout, making small talk and drinking their complementary morning coffee. A white South African man steps up to the podium next to a massive projector screen and begins to speak: "Those of you who were here last year, might recall we- we started off with a choir. Now it's become a bit of a tradition. So [name] has arranged for the Durban Hospital choir, the Thembisa choir, to sort of get things rolling and get us all into the spirit of the meeting. So, we'd like the choir to begin. Are they gonna s- are they gonna be at the back?" At that moment, Siphesihle begins the first song. The choir walks up to the front of the room as they sing, and they continue performing for about fifteen minutes.

The choir's participation in this medical conference has been heavily predetermined. This can be seen first in the physical organization of bodies in space and the clothing worn by the various parties. While other conference-goers wear the dress shirts, blouses, ties, skirts, and slacks familiar to many as professional attire, Thembeka choir members distinguish themselves as ethnically Zulu through their own professional attire. While conference-goers stand around in groups making small talk in the conference room, choir members find a secluded corner of the lobby to prepare for their performance and appear in the conference room only at the time they become performers on stage. These physical aspects of the choir's performance mark the group as outside of the main focus of the conference. Rather, they are an introduction or performative sidebar to the day's main events. The choir is supposed to enter, perform, and then leave, allowing the medical conference to progress.

The structuring of the choir's participation is also evident in the talk itself. The announcer speaks *about* the choir rather than *to* the choir, as seen in his pronoun usage. He states, "we'd like the choir to begin," separating a "we" (likely hospital staff or conference organizers) from "the choir." The announcer also asks, "are they gonna be at the back?" using the third person pronoun "they" rather than the second person pronoun "you" to question a third party organizer about how the choir would participate rather than speaking directly to choir members.

The most significant feature of the example for this discussion, though, is that the man who introduced the choir calls them the "Thembisa choir" and says they are from "Durban Hospital," even though the group severed formal ties with the hospital over a year before this event and the choir has renamed their group the Thembeka choir. At the beginning of his introduction, this announcer links the current performance to the conference last year, calling it "a bit of a tradition" to have the choir perform. He constructs a story of a partnership with the choir that had been forged years ago. When he says this, I am surprised. This does not fit with my understanding of the choir's separation from Durban Hospital.

After the performance I go with Philani to get some coffee and scones from the nearby lobby. There, I ask him about the misnaming. He responds under his breath, "I know, I HATE it when they do that! It means that they're taking advantage of us"; yet when I later review the video of the performance, I can see that no one in the choir even flinches when the announcer misnames them. It seems that the announcer does not know that the choir has renamed itself or cannot distinguish between the two distinct isiZulu names. Thembisa is translated as the verb "be promising" while Thembeka is translated as "be trustworthy/reliable." Furthermore, due to the power differential inherent in the Durban Hospital doctors' role as gatekeepers to other global health communities and the circulation of resources, choir members felt unable to correct them. It seemed that to this audience of global health professionals, the distinction between the words Thembeka and Thembisa was insignificant.

Transparency Report

Two weeks later, the choir holds a retreat aimed at reorganizing and remotivating the group (also discussed in chapter 8). They have booked a rustic site in the middle of a forest near Pietermaritzburg that is used for corporate retreats. A friend of one group member works there. We are staying for the weekend in a building that includes two dormitory rooms with multiple bunk beds, a common area, a kitchen, and a common bathroom. As we settle in on the couches in the common area, I mention the misnaming of the choir at the conference. In response, group members become highly animated. "It's exploitation, Steve!" Siphesihle exclaims. Zethu rushes to her bunk bed, rummages through her bag, and returns with a brochure and invitation for the hospital's celebration of the HIV clinic's ten-year anniversary. The brochure has been sent out to a number of the hospital's major donors and stakeholders. On the cover of the brochure there is a picture of several of the choir members, including Zethu, in their performance uniforms. The group is not mentioned by name in the brochure, but a letter inviting the choir to perform at this ten-year anniversary was addressed to "Thembisa choir." Group members are incensed. The appearance of their picture on the brochure cover adds insult to injury. The general attitude held by choir members is that they are being used for fundraising by the hospital without compensation.

It is at this moment, after nine months of participant-observation with the choir, that I first get a clear indication of the choir's anger and worry about their relationship to Durban Hospital. I am told that choir members began to notice signs that indicated to them that the hospital may have been taking advantage of them after they had collaborated with the hospital for some time and gone on multiple tours. For instance, according to the choir, one donor gave the HIV clinic money specifically to buy computers that were to be used for support group members to be able to access information about HIV through the Internet. The computers were purchased, but only doctors and counselors were allowed to use them. In the choir's version of this story, the perception of misuse of funds and the lack of appropriate compensation for their performances eventually led to a bureaucratic showdown: the Christian aid group organizing the choir's tours asked for a "transparency report" on the usage of their funds. The choir also asked for a copy of this report. When neither the aid group nor the choir received a report, both groups severed ties with the hospital. At that point, after lengthy discussion with hospital staff, the group changed their name from Thembisa to Thembeka to avoid confusion about the association of the choir with the Durban Hospital clinic of the same name (the Thembisa AIDS clinic).

This story is very different from the one that Chris, a white South African man who was the choir's former manager, told me in an interview I conducted with him. He said he did not know anything about a transparency report. Chris had been recruited to be the group's manager in part because he had previously been a singing competition judge (such as the ones in which isiZulu-speaking children would compete). His musical evaluation of the choir was that it was not good enough to succeed as a performing group without the help of the hospital and the impetus of donors wanting to fund HIV support and treatment. In other words, Chris thought that the reason the choir was successful was because it was an inspiring story about an HIV-positive group, not because it was an excellent musical group.

Chris felt that over time, choir members became more and more overconfident. As an example of this overconfidence, Chris told me a story about choir members' behavior on a flight to the United States. He said that on the plane, several choir members had walked up and down the aisle with autographed photos, attempting to sell them to random passengers. To Chris, this was an indication of pure hubris. When I asked choir members about this, they denied that anything like this had ever happened. Chris agreed that the choir had changed its name but countered that the hospital staff found the name change to be inadequate. According to him, there was not enough of a difference between the names Thembisa and Thembeka. That the choir did not adequately change their name was especially frustrating to Chris because the hospital had given the choir about 60,000 rand (9,000 dollars) for the legal rights to a CD recording the group had done, but the hospital had never released the CD.

It is impossible for me to say whose story was more accurate in hindsight. Regardless, Chris's version of events confirms that the choir had indeed separated from the hospital, that they had changed their name, and that they had informed the hospital that they had changed their name. In a national context where twenty million people spoke isiZulu, and in a city that was the heart of the province where isiZulu was spoken by the most people, the inability or unwillingness of white South African doctors to recognize a simple isiZulu phonological difference was striking, but not surprising. The implicit power differentials associated with global health functioned to reproduce patterns of racialized, class-based inequities that were common in South Africa more generally. Choir members' worries about exploitation were directly tied to the recurrent shape of the choir's participation in Durban Hospital events in the past and present. The structuring of the medical conference described in this chapter was just the latest instantiation of unequal participation by the choir in global health. As both Philani's question about the similarity among medical conferences and the introducer's assertion that "it's become a bit of a tradition" indicate, the choir and the hospital had established regular ways of interacting with one another. Such regular patterns were tied to both the history of the choir and the history of racialized inequities in South Africa and in global health.

HARMONIZING A CAPPELLA FOR GLOBAL HEALTH AUDIENCES

I had been attending weekly choir practice for almost eight months before the group performed at the medical convention described. At rehearsals, I often sat and observed, operating the small video camera I brought along. I also played my saxophone along with the group a few times. This was enjoyable and well received, but there was not really space in the music for jazz saxophone. I did participate, however, by helping to troubleshoot the choir's old, heavily used PA system (a set of large speakers and a soundboard that provided amplification for instruments and microphones). The choir needed the PA system because they usually rehearsed with drums, bass, and keyboard, and wanted to perform this way as well. When they were hired to perform at two medical conferences in late August and early September (including the one described in this chapter), they abruptly stopped using their equipment. Instead, they began to rehearse only a cappella choral music in four-part harmony. I learned that this shift was a response to directions given to the group by the South African doctors who had hired them.

"The Delegates from U.S. and All This Stuff"

It is late August 2008. At the beginning of their first rehearsal without instruments, group members stand near each other while one group leader, Siphesihle, explains the process he had gone through in negotiating their future performances, discussing the (meager) pay and the logistics involved.

Another group member asks Siphesihle what sort of music they will perform. He responds with a bit of sarcasm that the organizers want "traditional" music. This prompts a response (unintelligible on the tape recording of that rehearsal) and laughter.

About five minutes later, as they are about to start rehearsing, Philani turns to me and says, "Hey Steve! *Sinenkinga* (we have a problem)." He explains that the people who have hired them wanted only vocal music, but that all year long the choir has been rehearsing gospel music with instruments.

I respond, "*ayikho inkinga* (there's not a problem)." I mistakenly think that they are worried that they would not perform well without instruments. I insist that they could sing very well! Silence ensues. Without any uptake of my compliment, I continue with a question, "*Ngobani bafuna i* traditional music?" (why do they want traditional music?).

"*Ngoba* (because) the delegates from U.S. and all this stuff are not inter-ested in whatever music except the African one," Philani says.

Many audiences, especially American ones, tend to hear music within aural frameworks that essentialize difference and hear/view the world as divided into discrete cultural traditions. African music has been subject to the same stereotypes as those to which Africans have been subjected. In addi-tion to the generic stereotypes of Africans in animal skins singing without instruments or accompanied only by handcrafted drums, international con-sumption of South African music continues to be heavily impacted by the popularity of albums such as Paul Simon's *Graceland*. On that album (pro-duced in the 1980s, ignoring an international activist embargo of the Apart-heid regime), Simon worked with—or some have said, appropriated the music of—a South African choir named Ladysmith Black Mambazo that per-formed a cappella (without instruments) (Feld 1988).

In reality, South African music—even music considered to be traditional by South Africans themselves—has been embedded in global patterns of exchange and circulation for at least the past hundred years. Scholars have examined the resistance of, and cultural continuity among, members of the African diaspora in the Americas, Europe, and Africa. Around the "Black Atlantic" (Europe, the Americas, and Africa), music was important to resis-tance, continuity, and social transformation, in part because Europeans tended to view African music as benign. Black musicians were often able to circumvent the otherwise stifling restrictions on the movement of black bod-ies as they toured in minstrel groups (Gilroy 1993; see also Piot 2001). His-torically, consumption of global popular music also played a key role in black South African cosmopolitanism (Erlmann 1999). Jazz, African American civil rights music, and most recently, African American gospel and hip-hop are among the styles that have been popular in South Africa (Coplan 2007; Jolao-sho 2012; Williams and Stroud 2014). At the same time, artists continue to strive to produce music that sounds authentically Zulu or South African but might nonetheless be consumed around the globe (Meintjes 2003). Indeed, in postapartheid South Africa and around the contemporary world, essen-tialization of ethnicity and tradition has been mobilized strategically to gain access to resources (Comaroff and Comaroff 2009; Kuper 2003).

When American "delegates" visited South Africa and wanted to hear "tra-ditional" African music, stereotypes promoted by popular media and cul-ture may have led them to conceptualize the choir as being outside the fray of global circulation. These stereotypes impacted the choir's agency to choose their style of performance, upsetting group members such as Philani and Siphesihle. The irony was that the use of music to connect to international audiences—to allow for international travel among black South Africans who otherwise would not have had the means to do so, and to solicit donations—was a quintessential part of the African diaspora. Even as the choir re-enacted and transformed this part of the diaspora in their support and activist work, researchers and other audiences ignored the connection of these actions to previous global circulation.

AUDIENCE DESIGN IN STORYTELLING: INTERNATIONAL DONORS AND AID GIVERS

Audiences consisting of international donors shaped not only singing but also linguistic performances of South African patient-activists such as Thembeka choir members. Laura's TBL donor video, discussed at the beginning of this chapter, provides an overt example of something that happened regularly on a smaller scale among Thembeka choir members, when speakers would shift into genres of talk oriented toward relatively powerful global health professionals and international aid givers. One of the most common ways that group members and other patient-activists articulated their perspectives was in narratives in interview, documentary, or public speaking contexts, where their stories were framed as transparent retellings of past events. Here, also, group members' transpositions of HIV into global health contexts were constrained by imagined and actual audiences of powerful listeners.

Choir members had a great deal of experience narrating HIV to international audiences. They had gone on tour five times to the United States and once to England. During those tours, Fanele had been the group's spokesperson. She told and retold the choir's story to audiences of doctors, aid workers, potential donors, and others, while other choir members listened and possibly contributed advice on how to better craft that story. Siphesihle, Zethu, Thulani, Philani, and others had also been interviewed as part of two documentaries about the choir. When I interviewed choir members and when I heard them speak to international audiences, I recognized similar story elements that appeared again and again. In other work, I discuss how South African gender norms shaped the ways that choir members and others living with HIV narrated their illness experiences (Black 2013). Here, I examine how HIV transpositions were shaped by real and imagined global health audiences, focusing on two patterns in these narratives: (1) positive framings of HIV infection, and (2) turning-point narratives.

The "Luck" of HIV

Early in February 2008, before I have met the choir as a group, I conduct an interview with Bongiwe. I want to interview her to get to know her better and to start making contact with group members. At this time, I know very little about the group and thus do not know all the right questions to ask. On the other hand, because I know very little about the choir, I also provide an audience that closely matches previous international audiences that the group has interacted with—white, middle-class, American researchers and donors. In this interview, Bongiwe tells me her version of the choir's story, providing a window into how group members position themselves for international audiences.

I meet Bongiwe on her lunch break at the Durban Hospital HIV clinic, where she works as a low-paid counselor for children living with HIV. The hospital is located in a middle-class suburb near downtown Durban, with leafy trees and greenery overhanging the small side streets of the neighborhood. The location of the clinic is close enough to the city center to make it relatively accessible to working-class and impoverished South Africans, but it is located in a neighborhood where few people from patients' home communities (mostly the townships and informal settlements surrounding Durban) would venture. This offers a reasonable amount of anonymity to patients who do not want to disclose widely.

Bongiwe's office is in a small side building that offers children toys and games to play with, including an outdoor play set. In many ways the space resembles a day care facility. This is part of the counseling setup, allowing children to have fun and feel comfortable while learning more about their illness as they reach the appropriate age to be able to understand it (see Clemente 2015 on youth and disclosure).[1] We sit down in a medium-sized office adjacent to the children's playroom and talk in privacy with only a few interruptions from a ringing telephone and a coworker coming to get her lunch from the refrigerator.

I conduct the interview in English. In the interview, I learn that Bongiwe was raised on a farm in a rural area. While many other group members lived for periods of time on their family farms, most also spent significant amounts of time living in the township or informal settlements. Bongiwe, on the other hand, previously had very little experience with city life or city ideals of what was possible or acceptable for a woman. Describing the area where she grew up, Bongiwe explains, "It's a rural area, where, like, a woman is just a woman. The only thing the parents expect for a woman is to go to school, just for a while just to learn a few things—to write her name, to be able to sign for your, maybe, important document. But not as far as going to get a degree and do things and be something big as now I see other women, having been given that chance as I'm here in town." Bongiwe then describes herself as "fortunate" in comparison with others who lived in the rural area where she grew up, because she managed to matriculate from secondary school (in the United States, called high school). After that, she "just got married and [became] a housewife."

Continuing her story, Bongiwe returns to the notion of good fortune and luck when describing her HIV infection: "It was not luckily, but I think (????)[2] because now here I am. My husband got sick in 1998. He was working here in town. So he got sick, he came home sick. We were not sure of what sickness it could be." Like other choir members' framing of their illness in interviews and speeches, Bongiwe describes her eventual participation in the support group and choir as a turning point in her life. Bongiwe insists that she never would have had the opportunities that she now has if she had remained in the rural area, so that, in a sense, her HIV infection was a positive development. Anthropological scholarship suggests that support groups may promote narratives in which group members experience a turning point (Carr 2009; Shohet 2007). During that turning point, people state that they accept the vision of the group and experience positive change in their lives. Many contemporary programs and support groups also promote neoliberal ideals of self-maintenance and self-regulation (rather than government or societal support) (Zigon 2011). For instance, a study of the Treatment Action Campaign (TAC—a major southern African AIDS activist organization), showed that TAC turning point narratives often relied on the idea of luck and emphasized the opportunities and connections provided by participation in support and activist organizations (Robins 2006).

Bongiwe has in fact been a longtime member of the TAC, which may influence how she articulates her infection with HIV using the term "luck." As she continues,

That's when I started to open my eyes and see myself stuck in something—so-
called HIV—then he [Bongiwe's husband] got sick and I had to come over to
town where he was staying and working so that I could help him because he
was sick, to get to the doctors and to help and things like that, and fortunately
he got help here at Durban Hospital. So that's when I started to come over to
town and be around where I've seen things happening around the life of women
and things like that. Because luckily I had this matric[ulation], there was a course
here at Durban Hospital which was a counselor course.

In this part of her story, Bongiwe uses the term "fortunately" again and "luckily," explaining that she learned more about her potential through her experiences caring for her husband. During her husband's recovery, Bongiwe was
also diagnosed with HIV. Her husband started taking ARV medication, and
she returned to the farm. But she had become unsatisfied with that kind of
life, and her husband eventually agreed to let her return to the hospital to do
volunteer work. Eventually, she was hired as a low-paid children's HIV
counselor.

A few minutes later in the interview, Bongiwe tells me about how she
became a part of the choir. Joining the support group and choir is the main
turning point in some group members' narratives. For Bongiwe, it is a second turning point:

I just joined the choir, not because I was a singer or an artist or whatever. I just
wanted to be involved in anything that was happening. . . . I just got myself
involved with the choir. . . . For me, the choir, before, was just the people that
we were having—only support group members—that used to come together
to discuss our issues of HIV and things like that. It was my second family at that
time, because it was so different to deal and to cope with knowing that I am
[infected]. And so being with the choir and being around the hospital, I don't
know, it was kind of a healing process for me.

Like other group members, Bongiwe calls the choir her second family. She
explains that after joining the group, she began to be able to cope with her
HIV diagnosis. After a short discussion about stigma, I turn to Bongiwe's participation in the choir, asking, "So, tell me a little bit more about the choir
though. Because, did you go on the tours that they went on, or whatever,
or . . ." At this question, Bongiwe becomes very animated, replying, "Wow,

Steve, that was a change of my lifetime. In my *whole* entire life, in my *whole* background I never thought of myself getting into a plane. I *never* thought of myself seeing [the] so-called U-S-A. So, that was one experience I won't forget, and I never thought it would be something that I would see with my eyes and as it just happened, it was one thing—gee—it [is hard for me] to describe what it was like." Growing up in a rural area with little money, Bongiwe never thought she would be able to have the experience of flying on an airplane. An HIV-positive diagnosis and participation in the choir opened up a world of new resources, access to which was controlled by doctors, researchers, and aid groups.

Bongiwe goes on to talk about the tour (one of six tours the group would go on), again using the concept of luck: "Luckily, I went with the choir for a tour … it was a (???) tour when we were on the mission of spreading the message of hope, because that was the vision of the choir. And the hospital was trying to work on trying to show the human faces to people, and also give us [the] skill to be able to deal with our diagnosis as well." Many group members conceptualized their work with the choir as an activist activity. They were proud of their performances in the United States and the donations these performances had solicited that helped pay for the building of the new HIV clinic at Durban Hospital. Here, Bongiwe describes her conceptualization of the purpose of the tours: to spread a message of hope and show the human face of the epidemic (as opposed to statistics about infection rates).

Semistandardized plot elements, such as the notion of "luck," the turning point of joining the choir, the concept of hope, and the idea of the choir as a second family, all appeared not only in Bongiwe's story but in other choir members' stories as well. Reliance on semistandardized plot elements may have made it easier for group members to talk about their experiences with HIV in a context of pervasive stigma. It also provided a connection to international audiences of donors, researchers (including me), and aid workers who tended to value disclosure and valorize activism by individuals regardless of social context. As will be discussed in chapter 7, this was one of two dominant moral/ethical frameworks about disclosure that were available to choir members—the other being a socially oriented Zulu framework of *hlonipha* (respect) for family, elders, and ancestors. The availability of international audiences who valued activist conceptualizations of turning points, hope, and family likely played a role in the development of this narrative of HIV diagnosis, support, and activism.

Amahle's Story

It is July 2008. Amahle and I drive to Pietermaritzburg so that she can give a speech to U.S. Fulbright students who are staying in the city for a Zulu study abroad program. In her speech, Amahle—like Bongiwe—draws from semistandardized choir plot elements to tell her story. The Fulbright lecture is my idea. I have been searching for ways to contribute to choir members' lives. I know that a researcher who previously worked with the choir was able to arrange a musical performance or two for the group using his connections to the University of KwaZulu-Natal. I have a connection to a Fulbright tour that occurs every winter (summer in the Northern Hemisphere). In fact, I participated in this Group Project Abroad a few years earlier. The program includes homestays, intensive isiZulu training, and lectures by academics on various topics pertaining to South Africa. I wonder if they might want to hear the choir perform. I do not suggest a specific amount for payment, but the study abroad program leader nonetheless tells me they do not have enough money to pay the group. In general, choir leaders never told me what the choir was paid to perform (e.g., at medical conferences), and I never had the confidence to ask, but they did tell me that they were never paid enough to be able to afford transporting instruments to and from a performance. After dismissing the performance idea, the study abroad leader and I decide that one of the choir members could come and talk about his or her experiences with HIV. We agree that this could be a great learning opportunity for the American students, so I ask Amahle, who has become my research assistant, if she would be able to and interested in talking to the students.

At first, Amahle is nervous about the idea. She has watched other choir leaders give speeches, most notably Fanele, but she has never done this sort of thing herself. I think that she might be able to give the same sort of speech because of a "personal profile" she has written. At some point, the choir decided to publish a book with their life stories, or personal profiles. However, Amahle was the only one who actually followed through with the idea and wrote a profile. Previously, she asked me to take it and revise it—to fix grammatical errors and type it up. I now think we can use her "personal profile" as a template to create some notes for her to use in a speech to the American Fulbright students. Here is what I write in my field notes about preparing for the speech:

I drove to the township to Amahle's house at about 11 A.M., and then we sat and figured out what we would do for her speech. She seemed to be having difficulties so I said we would make it like a conversation, that I could help her by asking her questions. She had my revised copy of her "personal profile" that she planned to use, and also we took some notes for an outline of a talk about her life and her experiences with HIV and her experiences with the choir.

Then we drove to Pietermaritzburg. When she actually gave her talk, I barely had to talk at all. I recorded it on tape, so now I have three versions of her narrative, the one she prepared on paper, the one from our interview, and the one from the speech. Afterward she said that she decided it would take too long if I asked questions. I think she did a very good job.

It was just like Amahle to make a split-second decision in the moment of performance about the format of the Fulbright speech and to take immediate decisive action about it. This was one of many reasons that she was a great research assistant.

   In July, Amahle and I meet the Fulbright students and their isiZulu professors in a small classroom on the University of KwaZulu-Natal (UKZN) Pietermaritzburg campus. Pietermaritzburg has an array of wide lawns, historic buildings, and a sense of insulation from the surrounding predominantly white middle-class communities. UKZN Pietermaritzburg is the original campus of the University of Natal, established in 1912. The room where we meet is like many others on the campus, with an aging beige carpet, chalkboards lining one wall and windows along another. The room is furnished with large rectangular tables arranged in a horseshoe pattern.

   After I introduce Amahle to the students, explaining my research and her role in it, Amahle begins by asking the students, "Ninjani?" (How are you all?). She then continues: "As Steve has said, I'm Amahle Ngubane, all the way from [a township in] Durban on [the south] of KwaZulu-Natal. I'm HIV positive. I was diagnosed in 2001, in November. Then for me it wasn't easy but now I'm coping very well." Right from the start, Amahle sets her story up as a turning-point narrative. She distinguishes between "then" and "now," emphasizing her current ability to cope. Amahle seems unsure how to continue, so she asks if I have any questions.

"Yeah, we were planning to talk maybe about your life a little bit," I respond, "to give them the background, you know? Maybe about where you grew up?"

This is the only prompting that Amahle needs. She tells the Fulbright students when and where she was born, and then says,

> I grew up in a rural area in the south of KwaZulu-Natal. When I'm in the rural area I'm in the place where there is no running water, there is no electricity, and we were fetching wood to make fire or to cook. We were cooking with Zulu pots—maybe some of you know about it, [the] three-legged pot. Then we were using that pot in a one-room house, we were making a fire in the center of the room and putting the fire there and making the food for the whole family. We are . . . a family of seven, but two brothers have passed away . . . so in 1981, I was diagnosed with a heart problem.

Amahle articulates a picture of her early life for American students who had likely grown up in a very different way. From a linguistic standpoint, this showcases how narratives are not merely linear progressions from past to present. Rather, they weave together past, present, and (sometimes) imagined futures. Storytellers articulate discrete life events and place them in conjunction with one another in a way that constructs a certain kind of narrative logic (Ricoeur 1984). Amahle begins in the simple past tense, stating, "I grew up in a rural area." She then switches to the progressive (or continuous) present and past tense: "When I'm in the rural area I'm in the place where there is no running water," and, "We were cooking with Zulu pots." These uses of the progressive tell the audience that these were things that were habitually or repeatedly happening. Her accommodation to the audience can also be seen in the question she asked them: "maybe some of you know about it—the Zulu pot." By talking in progressive/continuous past and present tenses, Amahle sets the stage for future action. She also shifts into the present perfective tense to denote an action that has been completed, explaining that while her family had consisted of seven individuals, two brothers had since passed away.

Moments later, Amahle shifts into the simple past again, saying that in 1981 she was diagnosed with a heart problem. This leads to about five minutes of discussion of her heart problem and the ways that she and her family dealt with it. Amahle talks at length about her heart problem because her involvement with hospitals and medication was directly related to her HIV diagnosis. As she explains,

One day when I was going to collect my medication at [the hospital] for [my] heart valve, I told the doctor that I wished to check for HIV. Then all the doctors were looking at me amazedly. Why? What's wrong with you? Are you mad, or what? I said no, I just want to check about my status. Then they asked me what? Why? Because you are looking healthy and there is nothing wrong with you. I said no, yeah I understand, but I heard that people with HIV, sometimes they had TB, tuberculosis, some they're having headaches. And then I said, so now I'm willing to know what is my status about. Then they took me to the counselor's room.

Here, Amahle includes some activist messages. One of the things that choir members want to impart to the world is that even people who do not look sick could be infected with HIV. Others may have symptoms of unrelated illnesses (opportunistic infections that affect people because of their weakened immune systems). As Amahle voices her own speech and that of the doctors, she portrays herself as more knowledgeable and less stigmatizing than the doctors. This portrayal matches oral history research that suggests that iatrogenic stigma—stigmatization related to health care contexts (White 2008)—may have been common in the early years of the South African epidemic (Oppenheimer and Bayer 2007).

Amahle continues her narrative, describing a period in which she avoided getting her result out of fear for what the result might have been. Then she finally received her HIV-positive diagnosis. That evening, when she went to work at the bed and breakfast where she was employed, she went immediately to tell her co-workers, but they insisted that she was lying. When Amahle told her boyfriend, he advised her to keep her diagnosis a secret, but this did not sit well with her. She eventually decided to tell her sister, Zethu:

Then I told my sister, hey now I'm going to die. So I'm no longer going to do anything, so I'm waiting for my time to die. She asked me, you are going to die now, why? I said no, I checked. I had my results from the hospital. . . . I'm diagnosed HIV positive. She told me no, take it easy, I'm also HIV positive. I didn't have time to tell you that. I was diagnosed HIV positive the time I was pregnant, my sister told me. So if you are HIV positive, there is still life [ahead]. You can still live your life to the fullest. So now I'm going to refer you to Durban Hospital, where you are going to meet other people who are like us.

This exchange with Zethu was the beginning of Amahle's socialization into the perspective of HIV support: there's still life ahead, live life to the fullest, and if you're positive, stay positive.

At this point in her narrative, Amahle begins to rely heavily on the group's origin story, just like Bongiwe:

> I went to do beadwork at that time. Then while we were busy doing beadwork, the social worker noticed, I can do something with these people because I can see that they can even sing. Because . . . if anyone can start a song then we all join together and start singing.

> We [got an] invitation from [the Christian aid group] calling us abroad to come and visit them there. It was our first experience, at that time, we were so amazed, all of us, we said oh we were waiting for this time to come. It will be the first time for us to be on the aircraft, the first time for us to be in America. Because we didn't even think of ourselves being in America. We just think that America is the thing for only white people, or people who are having a lot of money, billionaires.

Like Bongiwe, Amahle describes traveling to the United States and flying on an airplane as transformative.

As a whole, Amahle's speech was compelling and interesting. She artfully crafted her story to transpose important aspects of HIV activist messages to this distinct audience. In doing so, she also explained her personal background and described the history of the choir. Amahle drew from a constellation of choir plot features, including the turning point of joining the choir, the notion of hope, and the idea of the choir as a second family. These shared plot features, developed over years of choir engagement with audiences of global health communities and individuals, both provided the tools for this unique group of people living with HIV to talk about the virus amid stigma and yielded a powerful framework for transposing their understandings of and experiences with HIV to contexts of collaboration and exchange with international aid groups, doctors, and researchers.

CONCLUSION

Across South African HIV/AIDS contexts, global health professionals were audiences whose expressed and imagined evaluative frameworks shaped how patient-activists engaged in global health collaboration. Shared biomedical frameworks and an orientation toward Zulu/South African/African culture as static, exotic, and homogenized, were key characteristics of global health professionals' "gaze" in their capacity as a powerful audience for the choir. Their positions as gatekeepers to the resources of global health privileged their auditory attentiveness and gaze. Experiencing the power of these groups, Thembeka choir members and other patient-activists engaged in practices of audience-design, transposing their understandings of HIV support, activism, and performance into these contexts. They crafted narratives and songs about HIV in ways that would appeal to global health professionals.

Global health audiences limited the ways that the Thembeka choir was involved in biomedical interventions. However, they were also central to the ability of the group to exist. Global health audiences shaped the choir's verbal repertoire in significant ways. In a context where HIV stigma was an ever-present threat, the ability of choir members to position themselves as being connected to such biopower yielded a positive alternative to stigma. Additionally, global health organizations provided the choir and other support groups with funding and medication. Patient-activists such as choir members existed at the margins of global health efforts, wielding limited authority and power as cultural and linguistic brokers for other patients.

This begs the question—Were choir members and other patient-activists marginal members of global health communities because they lacked expertise where doctors and researchers had substantial training? Or were they marginalized by the structure of global health institutions and interventions? My research experience suggests the latter (see also Brada 2017). It is true that if one conceptualizes the human body as a mechanistic object on which to work, doctors' and researchers' biomedical expertise is paramount. However, medical anthropology insists that humans—including doctors and researchers—are never simply bodies, but rather are always embedded in social hierarchies, linguistic conventions, and cultural standpoints for understanding the world. In South Africa in 2008, HIV patient-activists were the ones who had expertise in traversing the cultural boundaries between biomedicine, Zulu tradition, and South African social worlds. They were the ones with experience transposing English medical terminology into conversational contexts with other isiZulu speakers. HIV/AIDS interventions would not have been successful without the involvement of patient-activists, yet as the choir's experiences demonstrate, patient-activist perspectives were marginalized and shaped by global health professionals' practices as audiences—including practices of dismissal.

5 · HIV TRANSPOSITION AMID THE MULTIPLE EXPLANATORY MODELS OF SCIENCE, FAITH, AND TRADITION

One mantra of the Thembeka choir was to "live positively." In an epidemic of staggering proportions, with group members attending funerals nearly every week and watching as family members and friends succumbed to depression, it was amazing to see group members continue to thrive. The reflexive embodiment of performance in singing and joking about HIV played a central role in choir members' ability to reconstitute a bio-speech community of support and thus to live positively. Underlying these genres of performance was an orienting principle of hope. This was part of the choir's default orientation toward Christianity. It was not simply an abstract perspective from which to view and understand the world, though. Rather, hope was an embodied, reflexive process of patience, expectation, and healing that included visits to medical practitioners, such as doctors, faith healers, and *izinyanga* (traditional healers). In South Africa in 2008, there were at least three general healing systems in place—scientific medicine, (Christian) faith healing, and traditional African medicinal systems (Scourgie 2008). Versed as they were in the details of scientific medical perspectives on HIV/AIDS, choir members faced a challenge in how to integrate faith-based healing and traditional Zulu medicine with medical treatment. Group members used English biomedical terms almost exclusively in talk about HIV, whether choir members were speaking in English or in isiZulu. These terms indexed adherence to scientific medicine, and group members explicitly valued scientific medical explanations of HIV above all others. Still, my ethnographic observations and interviews revealed that choir members carefully navigated the interstices of scientific medicine, faith-based healing, and traditional Zulu medicine, transposing a narrow biomedical model of HIV across these contexts while simultaneously leaving room for other forms of explanation and healing for non-HIV-related health issues. I expected that choir members might have held language ideologies that closely linked English to scientific medicine and isiZulu to traditional healing, such that to switch into isiZulu would index explanatory models associated with traditional healing. However, what I found was that choir members transposed a biomedical model of HIV across languages and healing contexts.

In this chapter, I discuss how choir members engaged with Christian hope and faith, how they managed multiple explanations of illness, and how these actions were related to the transposition of biomedical models of HIV. In conjunction with shared language ideologies that both valued English biomedical terminology and linked that terminology with biomedical models, HIV transposition formed a central part of the choir's shared ways of explaining illness and seeking out care. Each individual choir member's engagement with the three distinct explanatory models was idiosyncratic, but all group members merged Christian faith with biomedical understandings of HIV. This was also part of how group members were able to simultaneously connect with global health professionals while also maintaining social relationships in their home communities. The practice of negotiating multiple explanations of illness was by no means unique to members of the choir. Many South Africans (and many people worldwide) engage in medical pluralism, drawing from multiple healing systems and cultural models of health and illness. As in other contexts, the relationship of these distinct healing systems to one another reflected and reproduced (and in some cases, challenged) broader socioeconomic hierarchies (Baer et al. 2003). Still, the choir's shared pattern of transposing AIDS—that is, insisting on the primacy of biomedical treatment in conjunction with engagement with faith healing and traditional healing—was central to the shared verbal repertoire that helped to maintain this bio-speech community.

In addition to research on code-mixing and translanguaging (e.g., García 2009; Woolard 2004) the discussion in this chapter draws from a long tradition of research in medical anthropology that applies the concept of cultural relativity to explanations of illness and misfortune. That literature focuses on detailed explication of people's understandings without (de)valuation or comparison with scientific medicine. Here, I discuss "medical systems as cultural systems," analyzing choir members' narratives in the context of ethnographic fieldwork to get some sense of their explanations of illness (Buchbinder 2011; Garro 2002; Good 1994; Kleinman 1988). I also utilize scholarship that focuses on witchcraft and its sociohistorical significance in southern Africa (Ashforth 2005; Ciekawy and Geschiere 1998), and I integrate research that analyzes Christianity as a set of malleable, globally circulating cultural practices (Comaroff and Comaroff 1991; Keane 2007; Robbins 2004). Finally, I am attentive to anthropological and philosophical discussions of the notion of hope as a Christian concept and an analytical lens (Barz and Cohen 2011; Crapanzano 2003; Mattingly 2010). A detailed analysis of the multilingualism inherent in Thembeka choir interactions indicates that uptake of biomedical terminology and models of specific illnesses may sometimes belie a more complex engagement with multiple forms of healing and spirituality, but that group members also differentiated themselves from other infected individuals by transposing biomedical models of HIV across health-seeking activities.

FROM MEDICAL PLURALISM TO TRANSPOSITION

Illness has the potential to create existential crises in which the "taken-for-granted" nature of one's outlook is challenged. When illness arises, individuals experience a break with their everyday outlook, and they will likely draw considerably from established cultural models in their explanations and experiences of illness (Desjarlais 1992: 137). The theory of cultural models is built on the basic anthropological premise that humans operate in a social world organized by publicly available symbolic systems that are to some extent shared knowledge. Such a lens for the analysis of human sociality emphasizes both the patterned distribution of cognition among community members and the variable uptake of cultural knowledge by a given individual within a community (Strauss and Quinn 1997). More recent scholarship suggests that cultural models may be understood as cognitive schemas that are shared (to an extent) in common among multiple community members (Quinn 2005: 478). The concept of explanatory models applies this theory of cultural models to the anthropological study of medicine, with goals such as the following in mind: "to understand how *culture*, here defined as a system of symbolic meanings that shapes both social reality and personal experience, mediates between the 'external' and 'internal' parameters of medical systems, and thereby is a major determinant of their content, effects, and the changes they undergo" (Kleinman 1978: 86). Explanatory models are often part of larger cultural models. For instance, South African faith healing is part of a larger set of southern African adaptations of and syncretic approaches to Christianity.

Biomedicine comprises just one set of cultural models for understanding health and illness among many, albeit a privileged and powerful set (Buchbinder 2011). Furthermore, individuals may draw from distinct parts of available cultural/explanatory models in idiosyncratic and syncretic ways in order to explain and narrate illness (Garro 2000, 2011). While American medical and psychological anthropologists have discussed these processes using terms such as "cultural models," "explanatory models," and "explanatory frameworks," the phenomena have also been articulated in other disciplinary contexts—notably including biomedicine—as "medical pluralism" (Baer 2011). Indeed, the term "medical pluralism" has become especially popular in recent years in applied health research (Penkala-Gawecka and Rajtar 2016). In this book I use "medical pluralism" not to discount the complexity of the phenomena as described in explanatory models/frameworks research, but rather in order to provide points of connection to biomedical discourses and applied research.

This chapter provides a conceptual bridge between this body of research on explanatory models/frameworks and medical pluralism, on the one hand, and research on code-mixing and translanguaging, on the other hand. As mentioned, scholarship on code-mixing emphasizes that in the context of a speech event, conversational exchange, or even a single utterance, shifts between languages are not random but rather are patterned. Switching, mixing, or borrowing may be related to pragmatic concerns, such as a change in a speaker's affective or epistemic stance, a response to other conversational participants' linguistic preferences or abilities, or an ideological association of particular linguistic varieties (aka codes) with particular value systems, institutions, or activities (Woolard 2004; Zentella 1997). Some scholars have suggested that the term "translanguaging"—rather than "code-mixing"— more accurately describes how multilingual speakers often draw multiple language varieties into a hybrid communicative toolkit that may or may not sharply distinguish between language varieties (García 2009; Reynolds and Orellana 2015; see also Woolard 1998). In Umlazi township in Durban in 2008, translanguaging (code-switching, code-mixing, and borrowing) involving English and isiZulu was ubiquitous—as it was in South African Townships more generally (Banda 2018; McCormick 2002; Slabbert and Finlayson 2002). Still, as the examples discussed in this book demonstrate, a distinct pattern emerged in research participants' use of English and isiZulu, rooted in a strong ideological association of biomedical understandings of HIV and English terminology. Group members usually used English biomedical terminology regardless of social activity or language (whether they were speaking in isiZulu or English). In this chapter, I connect this ideological association and speech pattern to choir members' explanations of illness and health-seeking behaviors.

HIV transposition was an instantiation of both medical pluralism and translanguaging—an instantiation that was rooted in biopower and bio-sociality. Biomedicine has developed over the past one hundred years to be endowed with a (perhaps) unique authority to describe and categorize human bodies (Foucault 1965 [1961]). This authority is linked to the increasing prevalence of biosocial groups—groups of people organized around shared characteristics or diagnoses as framed and understood by the authority of biomedicine (Rabinow 1992; Guell 2011). In chapter 3, I described the choir as a bio-speech community (rather than a biosocial group) in order to include an analysis of how language, particularly the embodied reflexivity of spoken and sung performance, played a role in the constitution of the choir community. Choir members' use of English medical terminology in reference to HIV was a key part of their translinguistic verbal repertoire (this is also discussed in chapter 6). In this chapter, I connect my analysis of translanguaging to medical pluralism, focusing on research participants' use of biomedical explanations of HIV and biomedical treatment within nonbiomedical healing contexts, such as consultations with faith healers. As mentioned, "transposition" describes how biopower and biosociality shaped choir members' linguistic practices and health-seeking behaviors. The term "transposition" models how research participants shifted biomedical terminology and biomedical explanations across healing contexts, and also hints at how the meaning of biomedical terminology subtly changed as it was recontextualized.

A Visit to Baba Shangane

It is May 2008 when I hire Amahle as a research assistant. She is unmarried, without children, and unemployed, so she has time to spare and welcomes the income. In addition, she and her sister, Zethu, have already welcomed me into their family, inviting me to their house and to their parents' rural home several times. Amahle has a keen eye for details. She is patient in answering questions about seemingly obvious topics (obvious to her but obscure to me), and she has an ability to take a step back from her own cultural standpoint to see things from a more anthropological perspective. Over a period of a few weeks, we begin to establish a pattern: on two weekdays, I drive to Amahle and Zethu's township home with my laptop, two pairs of headphones, and an audio cord splitter. We spend two hours transcribing and translating. Amahle does not know how to type, so we divide the transcription session in half. During the first hour, she types. This slows the transcription process down significantly but allows Amahle to work on her typing skills. This will result in her acquiring a new skill that will benefit her after I leave South Africa. During the second hour, I type. Often after the transcription session she, her niece, and her nephew (Zethu's son) spend some time playing with the typing program, "Mavis Beacon Teaches Typing," and we end up doing various other activities—eating lunch, going shopping so Amahle can take advantage of the availability of a car, or going to one of Amahle's friend's homes.

In July, Amahle and Zethu's mother falls ill. She moves from their rural area home to stay with the sisters in the township to be cared for by the family and to have easier access to medical care. One day when I arrive for our transcription session, neither Amahle's mother nor another of Amahle's sisters are at the house. A Christian faith healer, Baba Shangane, has asked to see her mother. Amahle asks if I can drive to Baba Shangane's house to pick up her mother and sister. Shangane lives in an informal settlement adjacent to the township. We get in the car and drive down a township road that takes us toward Siphesihle's house (where choir rehearsals are held). Amahle asks me to make a right turn into what looks like a dirt parking area for a small roadside pub. I carefully nudge the compact car up over the curb of the road and onto the dirt area. At this point, I notice a concrete strip that begins just behind the bar, threading its way along the edge of a precipitous hillside and around a corner. This concrete strip is not very different from a large concrete drainage ditch—perhaps it once was one. We follow the narrow road around the bend, and a different world appears. A number of cinderblock homes are perched precariously on the hill, surrounded by shacks constructed of corrugated iron or cardboard and tarps. Amahle points to a steep dirt driveway. "*Laphaya* (there)," she directs me. After a few skids and restarts of the manual-transmission vehicle, the car lurches to a halt in front of a small convenience store (a "tuck shop").

On one side of the dirt driveway is the faith healer's house. It looks quite substantial for a home in an informal settlement, with a large living room and a solid cinderblock construction with corrugated iron roofing. Next to the house is a partially completed structure made of two-by-fours and plywood. Upon completion, Baba Shangane's congregation will meet there. At the back of the structure is a finished room with plywood floors where Baba Shangane offers consultations with people who are seeking healing.

I never get to see the inside of that room. Baba Shangane never invites me in, and Amahle and Zethu indicate that the efficacy of his faith-based treatments might be impacted by the presence of an observer, so I decide to just let things be. Instead, I sit on a wooden bench running along the side of the house with many women and a few men. It is late afternoon, and children are playing in the grassy yard. Amahle's sister and mother are there (they arrived at 7:30 A.M.). Amahle's sister tells me that some people have been waiting since 5 A.M. Their mother's consultation is finished at 4:30 P.M., and I drive everyone home.

Before becoming a healer, Baba Shangane worked for a local newspaper. Then he "found his calling" and quit his job to take up full-time work as a faith healer. When people such as Amahle's mother go to visit him, they are supposed to bring a large bottle or bottles of water—several liters. Baba Shangane prays for them and blesses the water they bring, sometimes adding some substance that gives the water various colorings—light yellow or orange, usually. He then prescribes various uses of the water, such as drinking it, steaming it and inhaling it, or swallowing it and then regurgitating it.

I was surprised to find that Zethu sometimes visited Baba Shangane for the treatment of various ailments—I say surprised because my first impression was that all the choir members subscribed narrowly to biomedical explanations of illness. However, Zethu and some of the other group members combined scientific medical treatment with healing visits to Baba Shangane and other specialists. When they visited these healing specialists, though, choir members made sure that other forms of treatment never conflicted with medications prescribed by doctors. For instance, Zethu informed Baba Shangane not to prescribe the regurgitation of blessed water, because this could render her ARV pills ineffective (more to come on this). In other words, Zethu transposed a biomedical model of HIV into this faith-healing context. Such transpositions, and the corresponding overlaps in care and understandings of what caused illness, were not just intellectual but also embodied. Group members felt the steam of blessed water coursing through nasal passages and misting their faces; they experienced sore knees as they knelt for morning prayers; and they sensed the disorientation and feeling of drunkenness that accompanied some of the ARV pills that were taken in the evening, taken at that time to minimize the impact of this experience on their daily lives.

Witchcraft, Traditional Zulu Medicine, and Faith-Based Healing

Everyone in the choir had been tested. They knew their status. They went to Durban Hospital clinic or one of several nearby government-run hospitals to get updated CD4 counts. When group members' counts dropped below 200, they began to take ARVs. Choir members on ARVs were very serious about adherence to their ARV treatment regimens. In some cases, this was a family affair. Once, when I was visiting Amahle and Zethu's family farm, I shared a room with Zethu and her eight-year-old son. I awoke at 7 A.M. to the sound of a cell phone alarm closely followed by Zethu's son's earnest voice prodding her awake, saying "Mom, it's seven o'clock. You need to take your pills." At the same time, many group members engaged with other forms of treatment. Each person's approach was idiosyncratic, but choir members shared the idea that healing practices must not conflict with their ARV treatment.[1] Here I overview a shared practice among Thembeka choir members—the overt rejection of witchcraft, alongside the embrace of traditional Zulu healing and faith healing—and I discuss how each group member juxtaposed these understandings of illness with scientific medical models and the transposition of AIDS across social contexts.

Rejecting Witchcraft

There was one explanation of illness that all choir members explicitly rejected—witchcraft. This oppositional stance is comprehensible within a cultural context in which a substantial number of people considered witchcraft to be a viable cause of illness and misfortune. That witchcraft remained a cultural practice and explanatory framework of illness in southern Africa after the end of apartheid is attested to by a wealth of work on the subject (Ciekawy and Geschiere 1998). Some of this research examines witchcraft accusations and witch hunts, demonstrating how they are patterned in ways that serve political ends (Niehaus 1998). Other scholarship suggests that poverty, hardship, violence, and HIV infection lead to forms of economic and spiritual uncertainty that may lead to increases in witchcraft accusations (Ashforth 1998, 2011; Pfeiffer 2002). While choir members navigated multiple explanations of illness in their own ways, all stated one thing: HIV was not caused by witchcraft. It may have been the case that this vocal disavowal of the links between witchcraft and HIV was actually thought of as a way to ward off the possibility of witchcraft, but I saw no evidence of even tangential engagement with this orientation, nor did I experience a noticeable silence in this regard, during nine months of fieldwork. Regardless, a vocal antiwitchcraft stance was important to group members because they had identified witchcraft as a central source of HIV stigma. Going home (often to rural areas) was a common response to falling ill (Wickström 2014). However, fears about witchcraft and associated spiritual pollution made such a response impossible in cases of HIV infection, leading to the ostracization infected individuals and alienation of those individuals from important forms of care.

Evans-Pritchard (1937) was one of the first anthropologists to consider witchcraft as a viable cultural explanation of illness and misfortune. His work provides an early example of anthropological approaches to how people may simultaneously manage multiple causal explanations. At the same time, Evans-Pritchard distinguishes "belief" in witchcraft from empirical "knowledge" and in so doing reinforces a patronizing view of African cultures (Good 1994). This patronizing viewpoint on nonbiomedical explanations of misfortune has not disappeared with the end of colonialism, but rather persists in many biomedical contexts. Patients' pluralistic engagement with nonbiomedical healing traditions, if they seek out such healing, often occurs in the shadow of the distinct power and authority wielded by biomedicine (Baer 2011). In South Africa, I was told that many ill individuals visited traditional healers or faith healers before seeking out biomedical attention, in part because visits to doctors' offices were sometimes prohibitively expensive. Especially but not exclusively in rural areas, many South Africans combined prayer and faith-based healing with visits to *sangomas* (King 2012). A *sangoma* was thought to have the ability to harm people as well as to divine appropriate cures for sources of spiritual illness. In the past, some scholars translated *sangoma* with the derogatory term "witch doctor." Part of the expertise of a *sangoma* derived from the *sangoma*'s ability to communicate with the ancestors. And persons could protect themselves by speaking with *hlonipha* (respect) to the ancestors and otherwise maintaining a positive relationship with these ancestors, who were believed to provide protection to those who behave appropriately (Berglund 1976; Ngubane 1977; for a contemporary perspective, see Teppo 2011).

These explanations for illness and ameliorative actions were common in South Africa in the twenty-first century, often syncretically combined with Christian belief in the afterlife, to the point where they were sometimes considered significant motives in murder cases (Ashforth 2005; Comaroff and Comaroff 2004: 195). Whenever I went with Amahle and Zethu to their family farm, the sisters brought some sort of offering to put on the family altar (which included a Christian cross)—a bottle of soda or whiskey, or whatever else their deceased relatives may have enjoyed drinking or eating. Neither Amahle or Zethu visited *sangomas*, but a significant number of people sometimes did so—some suggest as much as 50 percent of the population. Often, *sangomas* were consulted in conjunction with scientific medicine. However, group members said that such perspectives on witchcraft and pollution contributed to HIV stigma. The idea that a person living with HIV might be spiritually polluted was incredibly harmful because it led others to completely avoid a so-called polluted individual. In turn, this might motivate people to hide their HIV status or sometimes to avoid getting tested all together. This was the opposite of what AIDS activists wanted. Instead, they oriented toward an ability to disclose widely, change one's sexual behaviors, and slow the spread of infections. This attitude was reflected in the choir song lyrics discussed in chapter 3, where *idliso* (witchcraft) was listed as one of a number of stigmatizing terms for referring to HIV.

When I interviewed choir member Celokuhle, she told me that she rejected both witchcraft and traditional medicine altogether. Like many other group members, Celokuhle was in her mid-thirties. She spoke English fluently, a language she had spoken growing up in the township rather than in a rural area. She projected an attitude of kindness coupled with an impatience for nonsense. I interviewed Celokuhle in September. Whereas my earlier interviews had been focused on learning the basics about group members' backgrounds and personalities, by this time in the fieldwork process my interviews had begun to reflect my interest in topics that I had identified as significant during fieldwork. One of these was medical pluralism.

It is September 2008. I arrive at the Durban Hospital HIV clinic and I am directed back to Celokuhle's office, a narrow space with a long desk and two computers. We begin the interview. After asking questions about her upbringing and HIV infection, I turn to the topic of whether or not Celokuhle ever visited a faith healer or *inyanga* (Zulu herbalist). Here is how she responds (interview 10-10-2008 in English, 11 min 58 sec):

> Um, well Steve, honestly, I think it all goes with belief. I just don't believe in such things, in such stuff. Honestly. That's how I was brought up, and my father used to hate this traditional—stuff, yeah. And that's how I ended up. I don't believe in them ((laughs)). That's the thing. Whatever problem I face—and there was once, there was a problem, I reacted to some kind of medication and my family was furious about it because they thought it had to do with something to be done like a *sangoma* and stuff like that, [that] it was witchcraft and stuff like that. But then I had to be strong. I had to take a stand. Because I just didn't even want to go there. I ended up coming to the hospital and I was admitted. Yeah, I just don't believe in it. Yeah ((laughs)). Well, particularly for HIV, I will *never*. Because I know what I have, and what to take if and when things go wrong. Yeah.

Here, Celokuhle strongly rejects the use of both traditional medicine and faith healing. She repeatedly uses the word "belief" to emphasize that she does not subscribe to explanations of illness that incorporate the possibility of witchcraft. She also brings up an instance when she had to defy her family's wishes in order to go to the hospital for treatment, rather than consulting a *sangoma*. She reiterates this rejection of witchcraft-as-explanation by stating, "Well, particularly for HIV, I will *never*. Because I know what I have." Here Celokuhle emphasizes her detailed knowledge of the biomedical model of HIV, specifically, explaining that she knows with what she is infected and what medication to take "if and when things go wrong." Celokuhle also makes clear her disdain for "traditional" explanations of illness, especially witchcraft and visits to *sangomas*. While other choir members were more muted in their articulation of opposition to witchcraft, all group members asserted that visits to *sangomas* were categorically not part of their healing practices.

Embracing Traditional Healing

While religious understanding and scientific understanding may sometimes be at odds with each other, as indicated by Celokuhle, this need not always be the case. In addition to consultation with *sangomas*, some infected individuals visited *nyangas* (herbalists/traditional healers) for treatment of symptoms associated with HIV. One choir member that I interviewed, Lethu, told me that he used traditional medicine to treat his HIV infection. Lethu was a tall man in his early twenties, over ten years younger than all the other choir members. He was a quiet, astute young person who lived with his mother in the same part of the township as Thulani and Siphesihle. These two older men of the choir had taken Lethu under their wing and encouraged him to join the group in part because the group needed a bass vocalist after Siphesihle and Philani began playing piano and bass guitar. Lethu often arrived at rehearsals in sports jerseys and a pair of sandals made from recycled Adidas shoes.

At the end of August, I asked if Lethu would meet me at Amahle and Zethu's home to be interviewed. Their house was the only place where I thought we might find privacy. Based on my familiarity with Lethu, I knew the interview would be a difficult one and that I would have to draw him into the conversation. Unfortunately, Lethu's soft-spoken interview responses corresponded with a malfunction in the old tape recorder I had brought with me. The malfunction created a terrible buzzing noise that masked many of Lethu's responses. This was a downside of traveling around the township with less expensive older recording equipment. Still, I managed to piece together some of the recording.

Lethu grew up in several different parts of Umlazi township with his mother after his parents divorced. At one point, when there was intense anti-apartheid fighting in the township between supporters of the African

National Congress and the Zulu-dominant Inkatha Freedom Party, he was sent to live on a farm owned by family members to avoid the fighting. As a result of being shuffled between family members, Lethu had gone to two different churches. First, he attended a Zionist church. Many sects of Zionist South African Christianity were derived from the teachings of John Alexander Dowie, an American missionary from Zion, Illinois (the term "Zionist" has no clear intellectual relation to the Jewish idea of Zionism). The sect developed in the early 1900s. Zionism has taken many forms, most of which are types of Pentecostalism. When South Africans talked about faith healing, they were often talking about Zionist healing (like the kind practiced by Baba Shangane) or evangelical prayer. Though this form of Christianity was introduced from the United States, it quickly took on a life of its own. In South Africa, missionary efforts resulted in syncretism with black South African cultural practices (Comaroff and Comaroff 1991). Lethu attended Zionist churches throughout his childhood. Later, he began going to a Shembe church. Shembe religious practices shared much in common with those of Zionist sects, but Shembe was based on the teachings of Isaiah Shembe, a Zulu man who claimed to be a prophet sent from God directly to the Zulu people. The church was more directly centered on a revival of traditional Zulu ritual within a contemporary framework and has as a result sometimes been characterized as being "post-Christian" (Cabrita 2014).

In August 2008 at Amahle and Zethu's house, Lethu and I sit down on couches in the living room. The sun is penetrating closed curtains, giving the room a subdued light. I know not to ask to turn on a light, because this would be a costly waste of electricity. I place my tape recorder on a glass coffee table and we begin the interview. Lethu tells me that when he was diagnosed with HIV, he first visited neither Zionist nor Shembe faith healers. Instead, he went to his uncle, who was an *nyanga* (a Zulu herbalist). I ask if such *izinyanga* were part of Shembe or Zionist healing. After all, both Christian sects incorporate a number of elements of African religions, such as speaking to one's deceased ancestors, performing ritual sacrifices of cows and goats for the ancestors, and carefully guiding the dead to their final resting place.

In Lethu's conceptualization, however, Zulu herbal remedies are distinct from those practices because they involve the use of medicine and are thus more comparable to biomedical healing. He explains, "Yeah, I had to take these things to make me strong. But what I'm scared of—you see when . . . I want to try this first. Finish with it. And then when I'm taking . . ."

At this point the terrible recording makes it impossible to discern what Lethu was saying. However, my response to his statement demonstrates that he was talking about taking ARVs after taking herbal medicine.

I ask, "Oh, so like, you don't want to mix them?"

"Yeah," he replies. In Lethu's understated way, this is all he has to say on the topic of HIV treatment. He indicates that the herbal medicine would make him strong. If and when his CD4 count drops too low he will stop taking the medicine from the *nyanga* and start taking ARVs. He does not want to mix the two kinds of medication. Like Zethu, Lethu explains that some treatments and herbal medications might counteract the effectiveness of the ARVs. Still, Lethu decides to take traditional medicine up until his CD4 count drops below 200.

Like some other South Africans with whom I spoke, Lethu saw traditional medicine as offering a first line of defense that might even keep him healthy enough to never need to take ARVs. Furthermore, as one lay–HIV counselor told me at a later date, some people thought that traditional healers were able to experiment with new medications in ways that were not allowed within the rigorous ethical rules of scientific medicine and thus traditional healers might find a cure. Though many people in the medical profession rejected traditional healing entirely, some doctors decided to embrace this logic, recruiting traditional healers and training them about how to identify signs of HIV and what not to prescribe as treatment. In particular, TB Leaders, co-led by doctor Laura and choir leader Fanele, approached medical pluralism in this way, and it seemed to work very well for their organization. But in all these efforts and health-seeking activities choir members emphasized that it was essential to prioritize ARVs—thus transposing biomedical models into these other health-seeking contexts—and to not mix multiple treatments in ways that would counteract the effectiveness of the biomedical treatment.

Hope and Faith Healing

One reason that nonscientific medical forms of healing were significant was that they reaffirmed people's faith, helping them to maintain hope. In South Africa, the Zulu root word *-themba* (hope) was ubiquitous in HIV/AIDS discourses (including in the old and new choir names). And though hope was oriented toward the future, it gave group members and others the confidence they needed to live positively in the present. Contemporary biomedical dismissals of faith can be traced back to nineteenth-century philosophy. For instance, the skeptic philosopher Friedrich Nietzsche suggested that religion was a kind of escape from reality, while Karl Marx famously called religion the opiate of the masses, viewing religion as a form of false consciousness that may restrain oppressed people from action. More recent anthropological scholarship suggests that hope pushes people's experience of time into the "mediate future," encouraging an ethics of expectation, constraint, and resignation (Crapanzano 2003). I disagree with these characterizations of hope and faith, at least in the ethnographic context of my research in South Africa. Whatever its ideological and imagined role in people's lives, I observed that for choir members, at least, prayer and faith altered how they acted in the present. Hope for the future, entrusted to an all-powerful deity, helped choir members to look beyond immediate experiences of stigma in ways that allowed them to go about the business of living their lives. I suggest that South African discourses of hope were ambivalently efficacious. In my analysis, the concept of hope in HIV discourses may have shifted public attention away from discussion of structural inequities that shaped patterns of HIV infection and access to care toward attention to individual experiences (compare with Fassin 2011 on "trauma"). In so doing, pubic discourses of "hope" were damaging for the design and implementation of HIV prevention and treatment. At the same time, though, for infected individuals, hope enabled action rather than constraining it and helped them to navigate stigma and illness.

When I interviewed Zethu toward the end of August 2008, I asked her about faith healing by bringing up the visits to Baba Shangane that I described earlier. Zethu was like her sister in many ways, but, whereas Amahle would spend hours carefully explaining the details of social events such as funerals and weddings to me, Zethu was less inclined to wax philosophical about her own cultural practices. She was a pragmatist. When I asked Zethu about such things, she would often give a brief response. When I tried to follow up on my initial question, she sometimes replied, "Steve, why do you ask so many questions?"

As with my interview with Lethu, Zethu and I meet at her home. The beginning of our conversation is strained due to the presence of her eight-year-old son—there are certain topics surrounding HIV, such as romantic partnerships, that I am hesitant to discuss with him around. After a little while, Zethu notices my discomfort and sends her son away, much to his chagrin. He is fascinated with America, and thus fascinated with me and everything that I do. I also think that the timing of my arrival in Durban, just before his uncle (the only man living in their house) died as a result of HIV, made him feel especially attached. But Zethu and I need the privacy to conduct the interview.

During our conversation, I bring up Zethu's visits to Baba Shangane. Figure 5.1 provides a transcript of that conversation. In this excerpt, Zethu is adamant in the face of my confusion that she does not go to the faith healer to deal with physical illness, only for "spiritual assistance." I wait for Zethu to expand on this on her own, but when no expansion is forthcoming I decide to ask the question in another way. She insists, "If I'm sick, I know that I'm just sick. Maybe I had the flu. I don't believe in those things—bewitchment or something."

This statement is very similar to the one that Celokuhle made about not believing in witchcraft. And, like Celokuhle, Zethu has had a lifelong engagement with scientific medicine. Remember that Zethu's parents had been taking her sister, Amahle, to the doctor from a young age for her heart valve problem, and Amahle had undergone a heart operation as a child. While Zethu did not go to Baba Shangane for physical ailments, Amahle once traveled to Johannesburg with a friend who also suffered from a heart problem. They went to visit an evangelical minister who was said to be a very powerful healer. However, like Zethu, Amahle insisted that her visit to the faith healer was only for her heart problem, not for her HIV infection.

During our interview, Zethu ends her statement by suggesting that there are some issues in her life that need to be dealt with. Perhaps I could press on with this topic, but I feel that I have already asked Zethu several questions about it and do not want to make her feel uncomfortable.

Instead, I ask, "and does that—does it ever conflict with going to church? To the Catholic church?" Amahle and Zethu attend a nearby Catholic church. They had taken me to a service to witness the opening of a voluntary counseling and testing (VCT) clinic on the church grounds. Though Catholic hospitals were among the first to open their doors to people living with HIV, the VCT center was a notable change from many earlier religious responses to HIV/AIDS that focused blame and responsibility on the infected individuals for their "sins." Responding to my question about using treatments from Baba Shangane that involve blessed water, Zethu explains, "I'm not sure. Some, they say it's wrong. But I think there's nothing wrong that we're doing because even in a Catholic church we have big drums with blessed water that

Steve:	Do you ever go there for things related to HIV?
Zethu:	HIV? No.
Steve:	No.
Zethu:	No.
Steve:	Just for other things.
Zethu:	Just for my . . . yeah, just for other things. Just for my . . . spiritual, yeah, assistance. Nothing about HIV.
Steve:	So, is it—I guess I'm not sure if I—I still don't understand with Baba Shangane. So you go only if it's like a mental problem, you're having a problem—or spiritual problem? But what about if you're sick or something?
Zethu:	If you're sick?
Steve:	Yeah.
Zethu:	He heals for health—people who are sick. Sometimes people come. . . . I remember the other day, other parents came with their child. He was a kid drunk. They went to Baba Shangane. He helped them. It was like a spiritual thing, yeah.
Steve:	But do you ever go if you are feeling sick?
Zethu:	No, I don't go if I'm feeling sick. If I'm sick, I know that I'm just sick. Maybe I had the flu. I don't believe in those things—bewitchment or something. Even though there are some things that it causes other people. But they don't make me feel—they don't make me sick physically. I can make it affect me in a way that, maybe . . . maybe find a man, you know. Those things don't affect me physically. I don't get ill. But there are some issues in my life, about me, that need to be dealt with.

FIGURE 5.1. Transcript: Speaking of Faith (interview 8-23-2008, 28 min 20 sec).

you can fetch, from my church, that you can use for anything in your house, you know? It depends how you believe. My church doesn't have a problem with those things." Despite the availability of church holy water for personal use, Baba Shangane is thought to be an especially talented healer. This is why Zethu and her mother visit him on occasion. And Zethu tells me that people visit Baba Shangane from all over KwaZulu-Natal, sometimes from as far away as Johannesburg (a six-hour drive by car).

The next question I ask Zethu is meant to focus our attention on her conceptualization of the human immunodeficiency virus. I had heard a radio show, an episode of *Radio Diaries*, that followed a young South African woman living with HIV who used the pseudonym Thembi (the Zulu name meaning "hope"). Every morning, Thembi woke up, looked in the mirror, and said "Hello HIV," telling the virus she was the boss. I explain this anecdote from the radio program to Zethu, then I ask her, "Do you ever do that?" She responds as follows:

ZETHU: *Mina* ((me)), I always tell myself that—and even if I'm talking to somebody else, even if I'm talking or counseling someone—I always tell him or her that you mustn't allow the virus to rule you. You must be the one who's holding the key. You must be the one who's leading the virus. Don't let the virus lead you. I always tell myself that I don't care about HIV. It won't kill me anyway. Something else will kill me. God knows what I still have to do in life. And since he gave me [my son], I still have, *ngisafuna uphila* ((I still want to live)) more and more, and see him growing, you know? I always—I DO talk positive with myself.
STEVE: Yeah. But not like, you don't say, "Hello HIV."
ZETHU: No no, I don't say that, but I always take it as a joke. I don't take it serious.

Here, Zethu moves into an activist/counseling way of speaking, perhaps imagining potential future audiences that would read or listen to the interview. She voices her response as a quotative, explaining how she talks to people when she is counseling them. She explains, "Don't let the virus lead you." In this sense, she is indeed talking of HIV as an agent—an entity capable of acting and producing effects in/on the world. Zethu then points toward choir members' practice of joking about HIV, emphasizing, "I always take it as a joke. I don't take it serious."

Zethu also highlights how her faith is significant. She explains, "God knows what I still have to do in life. And since he gave me [my son] . . . I still want to live more and more and see him growing."

As these moments from my interview with Zethu demonstrate, faith in general and hope in particular were important backdrops for the choir's activities and ideologies. As mentioned, the term *ithemba* (hope) appeared in numerous documentaries, pseudonyms of people living with HIV, and nongovernmental organization names throughout South Africa, including the name of the choir and the clinic with which it had been associated. And, after all, the group was a gospel choir. While commonsense public discourses of hope often view it as a human universal (something inherently human found across all cultural contexts), a closer examination suggests that this is not accurate. Even in the con-

text of the famous Pandora's box myth, the notion of hope changed over historical time as different Greek poets told the story (Adams 1932: 195).

In the sense that many choir members and many South Africans more generally used the term, hope was a distinctly Christian concept (Aquinas 2006
[13th century]; Augustine 1998 [5th century]). It *was* relatively passive, involving the expectation that God would sort things out in the mediate future
(Crapanzano 2003: 6; Minkowski 1970). Still, as in other therapeutic contexts,
Thembeka choir members' positive outlook was contrasted with despair. As
mentioned, it provided group members with an alternative standpoint from
which to gauge their actions in the present moment (Mattingly 1998: 157,
2010). Hope was part of an often-implicit narrative framework informing
group members' interactions which suggested that, with faith, things would
work out for the best. It helped group members to create a story of what was
possible that yielded a powerful vehicle for self-making (Ochs and Capps
1997: 87; Ricoeur 1984).

As a Christian concept, hope also provided a way to connect with Christian aid groups and other international audiences. Christianity has long been
an engine of uneven global circulation that has powered the movement of
people, money, technology, artifacts, and ideas across national and socioeconomic boundaries (Comaroff and Comaroff 1991; Keane 2007). Christianity supplies a constellation of cultural practices that often become laminated
onto previously existing ideologies and frameworks in idiosyncratic and
interesting ways (Robbins 2004). In contemporary (South) African contexts,
Christianity has also been a key part of how people from marginalized communities engaged with a near-constant flow of religious aid-worker tourists
who travel to various parts of Africa for "service" work. The choir's emphasis on hope and faith (indicated in my interview with Zethu) was not only
an accurate representation of their actions and orientations toward faith but
was also appealing to such researchers, doctors, and aid workers.

Managing Medical Pluralism While Transposing Biomedical
Understandings of HIV

Like many other South Africans, choir members were faced with a difficult
challenge in the management of these multiple explanations of HIV. Scientific
medical models existed alongside concepts provided by a number of distinct
Christian faith healing traditions and two traditional Zulu medicinal/spiritual

institutions. Choir members managed these multiple explanations based on their own beliefs and upbringings in dialogue with the socioeconomic, explanatory, and physiological power of biomedicine. What all of these strategies shared in common was a language ideological valuation of English biomedical terminology in conjunction with the conviction that biomedical understandings of HIV were valid, and medical treatment should not be contradicted by other forms of treatment. Such a conviction developed in the context of choir members' dialogues with doctors and social workers at Durban Hospital clinic before I met the group. This is not meant to diminish the agency of choir members. Rather, it highlights their creativity in incorporating biomedical understandings of HIV into their explanations of illness such that they were able to transpose HIV while engaging with multiple forms of treatment.

In interviews and in many everyday interactions discussed throughout this book, choir members used English and isiZulu terms to index a contrast between the objectivity of biomedical understandings of HIV (indexed by using English terms), on the one hand, and the potentially stigmatizing models of illness of traditional Zulu explanatory frameworks of HIV (indexed by using isiZulu terms), on the other. In this lexical dichotomy, faith occupied an ambiguous middle ground. A narrow examination of choir members' linguistic practices would have led to inaccurate conclusions about group members' health-seeking actions. While the choir's knowledge of biomedicine was displayed through their reliance on English medical terms and their general avoidance of isiZulu terms for HIV, group members' broader explanations of illness and health-seeking activities were considerably more complex. They not only sought out scientific medical care but also went to faith healers and Zulu *nyangas* (herbalists) on occasion (but never a *sangoma*). Linguistic analysis provided a solution to only part of this puzzle and needed to be supplemented by ethnographic inquiry, including participant observation and interviews. Group members found idiosyncratic ways to manage the multiple explanatory models of science, faith, and tradition, to explain HIV and talk about it in order to make life-or-death decisions about medical care. However, they shared in common an emphasis on transposition of biomedical understandings of HIV, attending to the ways that such treatment could or could not be merged with other forms of healing. An emphasis on English biomedical terminology and a shared ideology that valued HIV transposition formed key parts of the verbal repertoire and language ideologies of the choir as a bio-speech community.

6 · THE LINGUISTIC ANTHROPOLOGY OF STIGMA

It is May 2013. I have returned to South Africa for follow-up field-work. Much has changed since I left Durban four and a half years ago. Philani and Fanele are estranged from the group (more on this later), Zethu is getting married, Durban Hospital is closing, and Amahle has a boyfriend. When I get in touch with Amahle to arrange a meeting, the first thing she does is to take me to her boyfriend's place of work. When I first meet him, Amahle's boyfriend seems suspicious of me, but kind. He says something about how Amahle and Zethu are always mentioning this Steve character, telling stories about "when Steve was here," and now he is finally meeting me. He insists on hosting a *braai* at his township home later that day. He stuffs me full of food, and I talk at length with one of his close friends. This, I think, is a very nice way for him to assess my character while also being hospitable and welcoming.

A few days later, Thembeka choir members plan an overnight *braai*, and I am invited. That afternoon, I drive Amahle and Celokuhle to the supermarket and purchase large quantities of meat, *paap* (cornmeal), and soft drinks for our party. Afterward, Amahle asks if we can stop by her boyfriend's house in the township. Just after I met him, he went to a private hospital to have an ear operation related to a hearing problem. He is staying at the hospital, recovering, and she wants to bring some of his things to him before we go to

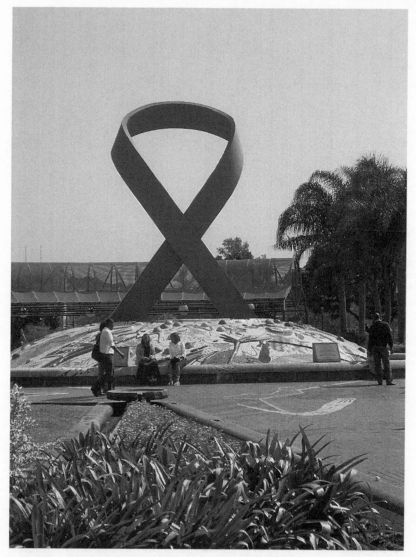

FIGURE 6.1. Gugu Dlamini Park. This statue memorializes Gugu Dlamini, a woman who was stoned to death by her neighbors after revealing that she was HIV positive in 2001.

the choir *braai*. She picks up his things, we swing by a mini-mall to purchase some sandwiches and toothpaste, and then we drive to the hospital.

Amahle's boyfriend is in recovery, in a shared room with one other man. He is clearly out of sorts due to the pain medication he's been given. Amahle opens her bag and begins showing her boyfriend the things she has brought for him. After a moment, he questions her about his pills. She shows them to him, then looks back at Celokuhle with good-humored concern and remarks in isiZulu that she is disclosing for him (*sengidisklosa*). I am not sure if Amahle means that she is disclosing his HIV status to me, to the other patient in the room, to the doctors, or to some combination of audiences. After this, we make our way to Bongiwe's home for the party.

Though disclosure is sometimes conceptualized as the result of a direct verbal exchange (e.g., one person telling another, "I am HIV positive"), in many cases it is subtler, more action based and processual (Clemente Pesudo 2007; Davis and Manderson 2014; Liang 1997). In the example of Amahle and her boyfriend, the simple exchange of pills became grounds for potential disclosure. Disclosure, even in these subtle terms, was relevant in that context because of pervasive HIV stigma. People living with the virus were sometimes ostracized, thrown out of family homes, beaten, or even killed. Indeed, in the early 2000s, even after a treatment of a single pill was discovered that would prevent an infant from becoming infected with HIV through fluid exchange during childbirth, some South African women refused to take the pill because this would reveal to others that they were HIV positive. In this chapter, I synthesize linguistic research on exclusion and markedness with scholarship on stigma, liminality, and taboo to outline a model of the linguistic constitution of stigma. I discuss HIV stigma in South Africa and analyze how Thembeka choir members responded to this with a distinct set of linguistic practices for referring to HIV—the linguistic component for transposing HIV. The availability of a positively valued biomedical framework for talking about HIV was significant in part because disclosure—being able to talk about one's illness and tell stories about it—had important mental and physical health benefits (Pennebaker 2003). This therefore complements discussion of disclosure and morality/ethics to come in chapter 7.

Little previous scholarship on language and culture focuses on the theorization of stigma (but see Goffman 1963). Rather, linguistic anthropologists and others often use terms such as "exclusion," "liminality," "abjection," or "marginalization" (e.g., Besnier 2004; Gaudio 2009; Hall 2004), while related work examines sociolinguistic markedness (Barrett 2014; Bucholtz and Hall 2004). Psychological anthropology, on the other hand, has discussed stigmatization at length, examining the individual and social-structural shape of the "othering" that plays a primary role in the constitution of stigma

(Corrigan et al. 2005; Jenkins and Carpenter-Song 2008; Link and Phelan 2001; Yang et al. 2007). This chapter suggests that to move from markedness and marginalization to stigmatization requires a linguistic theory of taboo (see Fleming and Lempert 2011). Classic and contemporary literature on taboo describes the embodied fear of contagion, disgust, and aversion that is linked to stigma, the ways that persons manage to refer to taboos without talking about them directly, and the ways that such aversion may be productive culturally and linguistically (Allan and Burridge 2006; Douglas 1966; Irvine 2011).

The analysis presented in this chapter synthesizes linguistic anthropological research on markedness and language ideologies with medical/psychological anthropological scholarship on stigma, contributing a theorization of the linguistic processes that constitute stigma as well as a discussion of some of the creative ways that persons respond to stigmatization. This synthesis suggests that stigma consists of the linguistic marking and language ideological construction of Otherness in conjunction with psychosocial aversion or taboo. The chapter also integrates research on globalization and global circulation into the study of markedness, exclusion, taboo, and stigma, discussing how the constitution of stigma and the creative sociolinguistic moves that Thembeka choir members made to face stigma were situated at the porous boundaries of social groups. Close linguistic analysis of ways of talking about HIV suggest that both HIV stigma and support relied significantly on indexing and marking the foreign. AIDS, like many stigmatized illnesses, has long been associated with what has been understood as conceptually Other.[1] If you asked an American where HIV came from, many would say Africa (Sontag 1989). If you asked a South African where HIV originated, many would say the United States or Europe. In both cases, people may hope to distance themselves from the stigmatized illness by associating it with a categorical Other. In isiZulu in 2008, linguistic marking through a complex noun class system played a central part in linking HIV with the foreign. Choir members, on the other hand, reshaped this association with the foreign. They allied themselves with economically and socially powerful Others—doctors, aid workers, and international donors. In doing so, they turned the Otherness of stigma upside down. Utilizing English medical terminology, choir members refashioned association with the foreign into a source of pride, limited income, and support. In this way, creativity emerged from abjection (see also Comaroff 2007). The positive ideological valuation of biomedical discourse, which was linked to engagement with global health groups, provided both an alternative to stigmatizing ways of speaking and a set of linguistic resources for transposing HIV across groups.

A NOTE ON THE WORD "STIGMA"

In this chapter and in this book more generally, I use the term "stigma" to refer to the social and communicative processes through which people living with HIV were marginalized, ostracized, or otherwise excluded from society. In part, I began employing this term because research participants (and South Africans more generally) used it to talk about fear, avoidance, and embarrassment associated with HIV. The term "stigma" was part of globally circulating discourses and was used when doctors, psychologists, and social workers talked about HIV. In academic circles, "stigma" has been extended beyond such specific cultural-linguistic practices. It is now a theoretical term and a unit of analysis, potentially cross-cultural in its significance. Recently, some anthropologists have begun to move away from using the term "stigma" because popular and academic discourses often view stigma from an individualizing and/or cognitive standpoint whereas anthropologists hope to emphasize the social, structural, economic, and historical aspects of this phenomenon (Kleinman 2012: 121). However, I think it is a mistake to abandon the term. Whatever else it is, the phenomenon sometimes labeled "stigma" is certainly rooted in individual cognitive processes and experiences. Also, and most significantly for this chapter, I think contemporary anthropological revival of the concept of taboo has much to offer theorizations of stigma.

The word "stigma" comes from the Greek by way of Latin, the earlier definition meaning a mark (made by a pointed instrument). Current popular understandings of the term are linked to "stigmata." One version of this word's etymology refers to the resurrection of Jesus. In this story, Jesus's hands, which had been nailed to the cross, retained the marks of those injuries when he was resurrected. The notion of marking, whether it is conceptual or physical, has been retained in contemporary usage of the word "stigma." But many entities and concepts are *marked* as being out of the ordinary. When people use the term "stigma," they are usually talking about something above and beyond sociolinguistic markedness. In the sense that I am using it here, "stigma" involves not only markedness but also fears of pollution linked to taboo. And more specifically, "stigma" describes what happens when these processes are applied to humans. This includes cross-species or cross-entity transference, as in the case of the historical stigmatization of Japanese people who worked with leather (Hankins 2014), or the stigmatization of people infected with a virus.

Erving Goffman authored a classic social scientific text on the subject of stigma (Goffman 1963). One of Goffman's most important contributions was his emphasis on the social, communicative, and, above all, relational character of stigma. "Marks" are markers of *something*. They are marked *by somebody* (Jones et al. 1984). They are part of social, communicative processes of meaning-making. Especially in the absence of physical marks (e.g., a noticeable physical disability or the wasting away of the body associated with AIDS), the fundamentally communicative nature of stigma becomes more apparent. The progression toward AIDS may include a long, dormant "stage 2" in which signs of HIV may be minimal. In addition, the wider availability of ARVS after 2004 in South Africa lessened physiological signs of infection among people who maintained an ARV regimen. For these reasons, among others, it is essential to understand the linguistic underpinnings of HIV stigma.

EMBARRASSMENT AND OTHERING

On February 13, 2008, soon after arriving in South Africa for fieldwork, I went to see a puppet show called *Amagama Amathathu*. This title was translated as, "a three-letter word." Popular media about the show explained that *amagama amathathu* was a common isiZulu term for talking about HIV (a three-letter word) without mentioning it outright. The show was being performed at an intimate venue in downtown Durban. Rows of about thirty chairs stretched backward and upward on risers, and a sound booth occupied the center-back portion of the room. The stage was simply the wooden floor, an empty space of about five hundred square feet. There were no props or sets other than the puppets, an aspect of the show's design that made it possible for the actors to easily perform at schools and community centers.

Deva Govindsamy, an Indian South African man who worked for the U.S. Consulate in Durban, had invited me to the show, most likely to help me gain some perspective on the epidemic and make contacts with other researchers, scholars, and performers in Durban. Deva was a short man with straight, graying black hair. Impeccably dressed, he held himself with the poise that was an important part of his job with the Consulate. *Amagama Amathathu* was a puppet show, but one where the puppeteers stood in front of and facing the audience, and so were also playing the role of actors. Though the audience was mostly white, people of many skin tones mingled together in a middle-class approximation of the touted "rainbow nation" that contemporary South Africa was supposed to be. In the front rows sat a number of black children who lived together at an orphanage. Their vocal, visually available reactions helped me—and seemed to help other audience members—to think about how the performance might be interpreted by children. The puppets were brilliantly made, with a mixture of realism and absurdity built into their design. The actors, obscured a bit by the audience's visual focus on the puppets, exaggerated their own facial expressions and tones. The show was a subtle mixture of children's aesthetics and adult themes. As the children in the front rows watched and listened, they laughed at things that I would otherwise have taken very seriously, such as people cheating on their spouses.

I later wrote down my impressions of the three parts of the play in my field notes. First, there was an older man who used his relative wealth to attract a young girl with no money. That section ended with the man going home to his wife, who then revealed that she was HIV positive—ostensibly as a result of the man's infidelity. Second, there was a "player" (an *isoka*—a man who sleeps around) who knew he was HIV positive. This man seduced a virgin, erroneously believing that having sex with a virgin was the way to be cured. Third, there was an Indian South African woman who thought that there could be no AIDS in the Indian community because no one talked about the illness. One goal of these stories was to raise awareness about how social conditions contributed to HIV infection and how people could ameliorate these through behavioral changes. The actors worked to combat the embarrassment and taboo that surrounded the virus through art and performance, much like the choir did through music.

Amagama Amathathu demonstrated one instance in which artists used performance as activism in ways similar to how the Thembeka choir hoped to do so. The play also provided a glimpse into a few of the key themes in South Africans' public analysis of HIV and HIV stigma (the significance of wealth and inequality to the spread of the epidemic, difficulties related to men's promiscuity, and reluctance to discuss how HIV affected nonblack

South African communities). The broader South African context in which *Amagama Amathathu* was set was also a "perfect storm" in terms of HIV stigma: there was the general culturally patterned embarrassment of talking about sex in public; there was fear of a virus that was not fully understood in a historical context of scientific denigration of black bodies that led many to distrust scientific medicine; and, related to embarrassment of public talk about sex, there were the confines of an age- and gender-based system of "respect" that prescribed linguistic avoidance of sensitive topics, such as sex and illness, in many social situations (Leclerc-Madlala et al. 2009). Avoidance and euphemism in any particular moment of talk, such as the use of "a three-letter word" to talk about HIV, could potentially be influenced by any combination of these cultural patterns that reinforced each other.

The Speech Play of HIV Reference

While I attended *Amagama Amathathu* soon after I arrived in South Africa, it was not my first observation of the linguistic patterns associated with embarrassment, fear, and respect in relation to HIV. That occurred when I interviewed Sthabiso and Lebo, two black South African women who were University of KwaZulu-Natal (UKZN) students. I first met Sthabiso in 2005, when I was in South Africa with the Fulbright Zulu Group Project Abroad. "Sthabiso" and "Lebo" were male pseudonyms that the women chose for themselves. While never mentioned as such, it is interesting to note that the choice of the name "Sthabiso" may have been the result of a clever combination of the word "stab" (a common euphemism for casual sex) and the common name "Thabiso." It is also interesting that both women chose male names. It is unclear if this was done as a way to point the blame for HIV toward men's promiscuity, as a way to further distance the women from the topic, or as a way to further maintain anonymity. I met the two on the UKZN Howard College campus in Durban. During apartheid, Howard College had been reserved for whites only. Its historic buildings rivaled those on any university campus worldwide. Those buildings were complemented by a beautiful hillside garden that offered spectacular views of the ocean and the city below. In 2008, Howard College was still in the process of merging with the Pietermaritzburg campus (described in chapter 5) and two other core UKZN campuses into a single institutional system. Each of the colleges had already been integrated racially.

Sthabiso and Lebo, both in their early twenties, did not clearly remember apartheid. Sthabiso self-identified as Zulu. She was a trilingual South African, speaking isiZulu, English, and Afrikaans. She had attended a multiracial high school near Durban in the mid-1990s at a time when such mixing in educational establishments was novel. She was forced to learn Afrikaans in school when she opted to take advanced math and sciences. The school administration had organized the classes in such a way that advanced classes overlapped with isiZulu classes, presumably in an attempt to discourage isi-Zulu speakers from enrolling in the advanced science and math courses. Sthabiso strongly identified with the postapartheid reemergence of a black middle class and was connected to international trends in fashion and music. This cosmopolitan orientation was sometimes in conflict with her connection to her family, who lived in a rural area south of Durban.

Lebo self-identified as a Twsana speaker of Ndebele ethnic heritage (two of South Africa's eleven official languages). Lebo's father considered himself Ndebele, but Lebo had grown up in a Tswana-speaking area. She had moved from Pretoria (near Johannesburg) to Durban to attend UKZN. Lebo told me how difficult it had been to move to Durban because she had been expected to speak isiZulu. In other parts of South Africa, especially in Johannesburg, vibrant multilingualism was the norm. While isiZulu was widely spoken alongside English and Afrikaans, there was no single dominant language. Furthermore, people's language ideologies supported multilingualism (Mesthrie 2002). In Durban, things were different. Many isiZulu speakers expected all black South Africans to speak isiZulu. In part, this language attitude was a result of Zulu imperial expansion in the 1800s and prolonged conflict with the British. Such historical events had led to a strong sense of ethnic identity rooted in the Zulu kingdom, Shaka Zulu as a warrior-king, and isiZulu language. Zulu identification was then reinforced by apartheid policies that encouraged Zulu exceptionalism in an attempt to pit black South Africans against one another. This was also connected to the recent commodification of ethnicity in contemporary South Africa wherein persons strategically mobilized ethnic classification to gain access to resources (Comaroff and Comaroff 2009). So Lebo, finding herself into a context where isiZulu was ideologically dominant, had quickly learned isiZulu, benefiting from the linguistic overlaps among southern African languages and the prevalence of isiZulu in urban slang in Johannesburg.

On the UKZN Howard College campus in February 2008, Sthabiso, Lebo, and I search for a quiet place to conduct our interview. We find an open empty classroom and walk in. I turn on my tape recorder. The room has the requisite desks, blackboard, and projector screen. It also has condom wrappers strewn about on a windowsill. "We call those *amajezi*," Sthabiso offers.

"*Jezi?*" I repeat. Sthabiso reminds me that *jezi* is an isiZulu borrowing of the word "jersey," a British English word meaning sweater or jacket.

Sthabiso explains, "They're just putting it politely."

"Yeah, you know, our language, and our culture, is very conservative," Lebo adds. "You don't talk about sex freely and you *know* you don't discuss condoms. Some of us can't say 'condoms' in front of our parents."

I suggested that this is perhaps not so different anywhere (I remember an extremely awkward teenage conversation with my parents about condoms); but Sthabiso and Lebo are not convinced. They insist that avoidance of talk about sex is of a different category than it is among white people, whether in the United States or South Africa.

It is true that the multiple levels of indirection, speech play, and verbal artistry with which young South Africans talked about sex could be mind boggling to an outsider. For instance, here is a scholarly explanation of some ideologically normative understandings of sex and gender gathered from interviews with young men living in a township:

> Within multiple relationships, there are two main categories of girlfriends, the "cherrie" (sometimes called the "makwapheni") and the "regte," as well as a one night stand, although this is less common.
>
> Regte and cherrie are both slang Afrikaans words. A "regte" is the "right one," or steady girlfriend, or "mother" or "wife to be" in English. This is the woman with whom a fairly permanent relationship is established, and often children are born from this union. The cherrie, or second best, is also referred to as the makhwapheni (roll-on, as in deodorant that is put under the arm, which is code for "kept secret"). Males say that they "love" the regte but that cherries are mainly for "sex that is fun," and each category of women is associated with different sexual behavior and norms. (Selikow 2004: 104)

I refer to these terms are "ideologically normative" because this analysis is based on interviews in which people tell interviewers what they say and do. The interview discussion is also metalinguistic: it is talk about how people talk. What people actually say and do may be another story, especially in the case of a group of young men talking about (or boasting about) sex.

01	Lebo:	no I don't know it. the treka term. and Hi [Vee is ((laughing))
02	Sthabiso:	[Hi vee.
03	Lebo:	another one.
04	Sthabiso:	and iHlengiwe Ivy Vilakazi
05	Lebo:	((laughing)) oh (what is it) =
06	Sthabiso:	= iHlengiwe is the H, Ivy,
07	SB:	oh.
08	Sthabiso:	Vila[kazi
09	Lebo:	[Vilakazi! ((laughing))
10	Sthabiso:	so they- they named it, Hlengiwe
11	SB:	yeah.
12	Sthabiso:	and what other terms do they have. I can't think of one.
13	Lebo:	yeah it's- I can't think of one ((laughs)). I think (they're quite ???)
14	SB:	mm.
15	Sthabiso:	mm.
16	Lebo:	people avoid saying H-I-V they would use. you know. other words.
17		slang.
18	SB:	hmm.
18	Lebo:	I think.

FIGURE 6.2. Transcript: How "They" Talk about HIV (interview 2-28-2008, 32 min 34 sec). Participants: Lebo and Sthabiso (black South African women who are University of KwaZulu-Natal students), SB (Steven Black, ethnographer), and a friend of the students, a study-abroad student from Holland who is observing the interview.

Like the speech play of the gendered sexual categories in the quotation about "cherries" and "regtes," my interview with Sthabiso and Lebo also includes some humor about sex. Some previous scholarship indicates that HIV stigma in South Africa is primarily due to the association of AIDS with death rather than with sexual promiscuity (Niehaus 2007). I do not see the two as mutually exclusive. In fact, the interview with these two women provides evidence of how reference to sex provided speakers with already-developed ways of avoiding talk about HIV regardless of the underlying reason for that avoidance (see the next section for further discussion of taboo). In our interview, I ask Lebo and Sthabiso how they talk about AIDS among friends. This leads to a playful exchange between the two students. The example in figure 6.2 begins in the middle of that discussion and includes transcription symbols common in conversation analysis and linguistic anthropology.[2]

In chapter 3, I wrote about how joking was a way for choir members to face stigma. Here, on the other hand, joking and play are significant in the construction of stigma itself. The two women go back and forth examining and sharing different terms that are used to talk about HIV, rather than mentioning it outright in English or in isiZulu. This exchange begins with Lebo stating that she does not know "the treka term," a term that Sthabiso has just introduced. Sthabiso has explained that the "tre" in "treka" comes from slang for the number three; and "three" referred to the Z3, a model of BMW car that was popular in South Africa in 2008; and the Z3 was fast, and flashy— in other words, it "got around." Note also that this was a European car, part of the association of many terms for HIV with the foreign (discussed later in the chapter). So when someone said, "uyatreka" (he/she is threeing or trekking), they were indicating that the person being referred to was fast sexually, was sleeping around, and had become infected with HIV. The number three also indexes the three letters of HIV (as in amagama amathathu "a three-letter word"), an association that was so common that simply raising three fingers had become a conventionalized gesture for HIV reference (Brookes 2011).

In line 01 of the excerpt, after stating that she does not know the treka term, Lebo introduces the term "Hi vee," laughing as she says this. Hi vee is a simple form of speech play, combining the "H" and "I" of HIV into "hi" and speaking the name of the letter "V." Lebo's laughter signals that speech play. In the transcript, the left brackets in lines 01 and 02 represent overlap. In other words, Sthabiso chimes in with "Hi Vee" while Lebo is still saying "Hi Vee." Some might think that Sthabiso is "interrupting." Conversation analysts, linguistic anthropologists, and sociolinguists try to avoid this sort of value judgment— thus the term "overlap." In fact, in this instance Sthabiso is engaging in what is called "recognitional overlap." This happens when a person overlaps at the moment that they *recognize* the word or phrase being uttered by another (Jefferson 1984). In some cultural contexts, recognitional overlap is a signal that the other person is engaged and paying close attention to the conversation and is not considered an interruption. This is what was happening here. Lebo and Sthabiso's engagement and excitement continues: the equals signs at the end of line 05 and the beginning of line 06 represent one person starting to talk at precisely the moment another stops talking; the brackets in lines 08 and 09 represent another (recognitional) overlap; and laughter is represented in lines 09 and 13. All of these moments of talk represented in the transcript indicate that the two women are closely conversationally synchronized with one another. They are "on the same page." Sthabiso and Lebo also introduces one other term for HIV, iHlengiwe Ivy Vilakazi, turning the three letters of HIV into the initials of a person's name. I will return to this term later in the chapter.

While I begin this part of the interview by asking the two women, "how do *you* talk about HIV," Lebo and Sthabiso end by generalizing how "people" talk about HIV. Their change in pronouns begins in lines 10 and 12, with Sthabiso saying, "so *they* named it"; and then, "what other terms do *they* have?" Lebo follows suit, using the general pronoun "people" and the third person pronoun "they" again, explaining "*people* would avoid saying H-I-V. *They* would use, you know, other words. Slang." Such a shift may simply be an effect of the interview context—maybe Sthabiso and Lebo think that they should be speaking in general terms as cultural experts about South Africa. However, it is difficult not to interpret this as a way for the two women to use pronouns to distance themselves from either the social action of using the terms or the feeling that they might be stigmatized as a result of just uttering the words. Indeed, across cultures metalinguistic utterances (especially talk about how *others* talk) has been noted as a key feature in the linguistic constitution of taboo (Irvine 2011).

Stigma and Taboo

My analysis of the linguistic and sociocultural contours of these and other ways of talking about HIV in South Africa suggests that stigma, in the sense of the term used by psychological and medical anthropologists, is similar to but distinct from other phenomena studied by anthropologists, such as taboo, sociolinguistic markedness, and liminality. Scholars conducting research on HIV in South Africa have examined the links between HIV, taboo, and (spiritual) pollution (e.g., Ashforth 2005; Niehaus 2007; McNeil 2011). Building on this scholarship, here I discuss the role of sociolinguistic markedness—in particular, the marking of a category of person—in the constitution of stigma. This model provides a way to connect stigma to the study of sociolinguistic identity marking more generally.

The concept of taboo became popular in academic circles in the early 1900s. Anthropologists, psychologists (notably including Sigmund Freud), and other social scientists appropriated the Polynesian word *tabu*. In Polynesia, *tabu* meant something broadly similar to the Greek *stigma*, translated

as, "marked thoroughly," with a secondary meaning of being sacred or pro-
hibited (Steiner 1956). Early anthropologists describe a relationship between
the maintenance of cultural and linguistic taboos and the reproduction of
social structures over multiple generations of community members. Mary
Douglas, a British anthropologist working in the middle to late twentieth
century, wrote extensively about issues related to taboo. In 1966, she wrote
what is perhaps her best-known work, *Purity and Danger: An Analysis of
Pollution and Taboo*. Douglas begins her book by critiquing the conceptual
opposition between primitive and civilized, stating that all religions are
"inextricably confused with defilement and hygiene" (Douglas 1966: 1). She
analyzes the prohibitions of the book of Leviticus in the Old Testament,
especially those that led to the Jewish classification of certain foods as
kosher (for instance, there is a prohibition or taboo of eating pork, ostensibly
because pigs have cloven hooves). Douglas argues that, like taboos identified
in other cultural contexts, these biblical prohibitions accomplish five tasks:
(1) the reduction of ambiguity ("by settling for one or other interpretation"); (2) physical control of anomaly; (3) strengthening of the definitions
to which taboo entities do not conform; (4) labeling of anomalous events
as dangerous; and (5) making ambiguous symbols available for use in ritual
("to enrich meaning or to call attention to other levels of existence")
(Douglas 1966: 40–41). Drawing from the anthropological theory of struc-
turalism, Douglas notes that religions in general, and taboos in particular,
create conceptual order by naming opposites, exaggerating differences
between them, and creating taboos for entities that do not fit in with these
conceptual opposites.

Some of Douglas's core observations still ring true and are helpful for
understanding HIV in South Africa and for conceptualizing linguistic exclusion in general. For instance, Fraser McNeill (2011) argues that "blood, dirt/
pollution, sexually transmitted infections, 'deviant' behavior, and medical
science have been strung together to provide historically constituted explanations for HIV under the wider 'folk' cosmological concept of *malwadze dza
vhafumakadzi* (the illnesses/sickness of women)" (179). More generally, too,
multiple examples from more recent ethnographic literature demonstrate the
significance of stigma (and taboo) in social spaces where a particular group
of people do not fit hegemonic norms associated with social reproduction
(Besnier 2004; Gaudio 2009; Hall and O'Donovan 1996; see also Black 2018).
This insight can also be applied to the case of HIV in South Africa. HIV came

into public awareness as a South African problem just as the minority-ruled apartheid government was being dismantled. The social and economic instability of this transition to a democratic government helped to produce what some have called "spiritual insecurity" (Ashforth 2011). Furthermore, AIDS did not match conventional categories of illness. As an autoimmune disorder, it manifested itself through opportunistic infections, and scientific studies were still working to find effective treatments in the late 1990s and early 2000s. Especially in popular discourses, clear information about HIV was hard to come by. In the United States and Europe, the virus had already been erroneously labeled a "gay disease" transmitted by homosexual males (Treichler 1987). HIV was also correlated with structural instabilities of post-apartheid South Africa that threatened the viability of previously "normal" long-term heterosexual partnerships, part of a political economy of sex that encouraged short-term relationships and multiple partners (Hunter 2007, 2010). Finally, people living with HIV were sometimes seen as being "dead before dying," and thus in a betwixt-and-between stage (Niehaus 2007). In these and other ways, HIV/AIDS did not "fit" into established categories. This made the illness a prime candidate for taboo.

LINGUISTIC MARKEDNESS AND AVOIDANCE

South African terms for referring to HIV relied on both markedness and avoidance—the latter being a correlate of taboo, of fears of pollution and inadvertent infection due to understandings about how HIV is transmitted. Amid "salient silences," gossip and rumor constructed AIDS as a social danger (Stadler 2003). One famous story of avoidance and fear of pollution involved former president and antiapartheid leader Nelson Mandela. Mandela was on a visit to a township in Johannesburg when he noticed a house that everybody seemed to be avoiding. He asked why. He was told it was because the children in the family were infected with HIV. Dismissing people's fears, Mandela went and visited with the children. When he came back outside, no one would go near him. He was forced to end his tour early and return to his limousine. Not even a hero such as Mandela was immune to the effects of HIV stigma (Ashforth 2005: 155).

The taboo of HIV stigma is linguistically constituted through the process of markedness. The theory of markedness was first developed by a group of

Russian linguists (sometimes called the "Prague circle") in the first half of the twentieth century. The core idea is rooted in the observation that some linguistic forms (words, phrases, or parts of words) are default (or unmarked) forms, whereas other linguistic forms include additional linguistic features that "mark" that form as different (Jakobson 1990; Trubetzkoy 1969 [1939]). Markedness is created through opposition. Sounds, words, and grammatical patterns gain meaning through opposition to others. Opposition is part of the patterning of all aspects of language. Here, the addition of a mark may reveal important assumptions about social roles and cultural patterns. However, these sorts of linguistic patterns are not just reflections of cultural biases, categories, and identities. They constitute them and reproduce them in interaction, as the unmarked emerges in social encounters (Barrett 2014; Bucholtz and Hall 2005).

Sociolinguistic markedness played an important role in constituting HIV stigma in South Africa. Figure 6.3 provides some examples of terms people used to refer to HIV/AIDS, including some that have already appeared in the book. These are drawn from recorded data and popular media (magazines, pamphlets, TV shows, and Internet sites). The first two terms are often suggested to be translations of HIV and TB, though, as discussed earlier in the book, they are not neutral biomedical translations. Each of the other terms involves speech play and indirection. *Amagama amathathu* and iHlengiwe Ivy Vilakazi (discussed earlier) both play with the acronym H-I-V. *iSlim* refers to the emaciated look of some infected individuals prior to the introduction of ARVs. *Umashayabhuqe* refers to HIV metaphorically as a person who abuses or beats up others. Finally, *iqhoks* involves onomatopoeia. The "q" in *umashayabhuqe* and *iqhoks* represents a palato-alveolar click. isiZulu and several other Nguni languages utilize click sounds as consonants. In *iqhoks*, the click consonant "q" and the vowel "o" together make the sound of high heels striking on a hard surface ("qho"). Using this onomatopoetic word for high heels as a term for HIV/AIDS only makes sense if a person makes the following connections: first, an association of high-heeled shoes with femininity, specifically a contemporary or "Western" femininity; second, an association of "Western" femininity with a negative evaluation of feminine sexual freedom; and third, an association of ("Western") feminine sexual freedom with the spread of HIV/AIDS through intimate heterosexual encounters (see Clark 2006). The gendered indexical links between *iqhoks* and HIV thus involve threefold indirectness.

IsiZulu Term	English Translation
ingculazi	HIV/AIDS
isifo sofuba	Tuberculosis (lit. sickness of the chest)
amagama amathathu	A three-letter word (refers to HIV acronym's three letters)
iHlengiwe Ivy Vilakazi	(Common isiZulu name made from the HIV acronym)
iSlim	Slim (refers to the wasting away of the body)
umashayabhuqe	The one who beats people up
iqhoks	High heeled shoes

FIGURE 6.3. isiZulu Terms for HIV/AIDS.

Many of the ways that South Africans avoided direct reference to HIV were also tied to Zulu traditions of *hlonipha*. There was great variability across communities and across gender, class, and urban/rural distinctions in how individuals practiced respect, but, as mentioned, many persons saw respect as a key part of being Zulu (Appalraju and de Kadt 2002; Rudwick 2008). Sometimes, people explained their avoidance of direct reference to HIV, especially direct reference to people living with HIV, as a form of *hlonipha* respect for infected individuals' privacy and the standing of infected individuals' families (Wood and Lambert 2008). However, as described in earlier chapters, the motivation to act with *hlonipha* was also linked to fears of spiritual pollution and subsequent illness that might occur if one did not enact culturally appropriate respect. In this way, speech play and alternative reference were central to the reproduction of a taboo avoidance of HIV/AIDS.

MARKING THROUGH NOUN CLASSES

In addition to speech play and symbolic valences, four of the aforementioned terms also share a particular grammatical feature that marks HIV/AIDS. Like many other southern African languages, isiZulu is a noun class language. In contemporary isiZulu, every noun is accompanied by a specific affix (in this case, a prefix). Four of the aforementioned terms include one of two particular isiZulu noun class prefixes: noun classes 5 (*i[li]*) or 6 (*ama*), which nearly always occur in isiZulu as binary choices for the singular and plural of a set of nouns. For instance, the singular *ikati* (cat) is matched with the plural

(A) *iyagijima*		"it [the dog] is running"		*inja* = dog	
i-	ya-	gijima		in-	ja
nc9-	pres-	run		n9-	dog
(B) *liyagijima*		"it [the cat] is running"		*ikati* = cat	
li-	ya-	gijima		i-	kati
nc5-	pres-	run		n5-	cat

FIGURE 6.4.   isiZulu Noun Classes in Action.

amakati (cats). Verbs must agree, grammatically, with the nouns of a sentence through the inclusion of a verbal affix that corresponds with the noun class affix. Every time a verbal phrase is uttered it must include an affix to indicate the noun associated with it. For instance, the phrase "it is running" will be different depending on whether it is a dog (*inja*—noun class 9) or a cat (*ikati*—noun class 5) that is doing the running (see figure 6.4).

In figure 6.4, both (A) and (B) include "-*ya*," the present-tense affix, and "*gijima*," the verb stem translated as "to run." The linguistic construction in (A) also includes the verbal noun class marker "*i-*" indicating that the entity doing the running is of noun class 9—in this case, a dog. The linguistic construction in (B) also includes the verbal noun class marker "*li-*" indicating that the entity doing the running is of noun class 5—in this case, a cat.

Figure 6.5 is a chart that shows all the noun classes employed in contemporary isiZulu. There are separate noun classes for singular and plural. Linguists assign the numbers used in this chart according to proposed similarities to other African languages of the same language family. For this reason, there are no isiZulu noun classes 12 or 13, but these noun classes appear in other African languages. There are two aspects of isiZulu noun classes that are significant for this chapter. First, noun classes make it possible to precisely control indirection and ambiguity. There are thirteen noun classes. This means that there are also thirteen distinct pronominal groups in addition to others for first person, second person, and third person singular and plural that could be used in a conversation. Given the right conversational context, one could speak about a topic such as HIV/AIDS without ever mentioning it outright simply by using one of the thirteen noun class pronouns that corresponded to the term being discussed. True, one can perform this kind of indirection in English as well, but there is much less specificity in the pronoun "it" than there is in an "it" pronoun equivalent that specifies one of thirteen noun classes.

Noun Class	Example (Translation)	Noun Class	Example (Translation)
1. um(u)-	*umuntu* (person)	2. aba-	*abantu* (people)
1a. u-	*uthisha* (teacher)	2a. o-	*othisha* (teachers)
3. um(u)-	*umuthi* (tree/ medicine)	4. imi-	*imithi* (trees)
5. i(li)-	*igama* (word/ letter)	6. ama-	*amagama* (words/ letters)
7. isi-	*isikole* (school)	8. izi-	*izikole* (schools)
9. in-/ im-	*inyanga* (herbalist/ moon)	10. izin- izim-	*izinyanga* (herbalists/ moons)
11. u(lu)-	*unwele* (hair)		* takes class 10 in plural form
14. ubu-	*ubuntu* (humanity)		* abstract nouns (no plural)
15. uku-	*ukucula* (to sing)		* verbal nouns (infinitives—no plural)

FIGURE 6.5. isiZulu Noun Class Prefixes and Examples.

Second, there is a limited logic to the categories imposed by these noun classes. Perhaps at one point in the past, the noun classes of Nguni languages parsed human understanding more fully into bits and pieces. In contemporary isiZulu, though, noun classes are, on the whole, grammatical categories rather than conceptual categories. There are a few exceptions, though—what linguists describe as limited semantic productivity. Noun classes 1 and 2 are often used for human referents including all personal names, and noun classes 5 and 6 are often used when borrowing nouns from other languages (Demuth 2000). In the context of noun classes 1/2 and 5/6, isiZulu is similar to other languages where noun class affixes "become the representative points of mutual opposition . . . the fundamental 'kinds of things' for the speakers of a language, who map such total partition structures onto many other realms of experience as a language- and culture-specific set of 'metaphors' by analogy" (Silverstein 1986: 504; see also Lucy 2000: 335). Among isiZulu speakers, not all borrowed words are prefixed with noun classes 5 and 6. Furthermore, not all words that are prefixed with noun classes 5 and 6 are borrowed. Still, in 2008 isiZulu speakers typically used two noun class prefixes 5 and 6 (*i-* and *ama-*) for reference to foreign entities and used these noun classes when code-mixing and creating new borrowings of English words.

Connecting this understanding of isiZulu noun classes to the four words for HIV/AIDS that take noun classes 5 and 6, I suggest that the use of noun classes 5 and 6 for foreign reference was recursively laminated onto HIV reference in popular discourse to index HIV/AIDS as foreign. It is not coincidental that many terms for HIV/AIDS were prefixed with noun classes 5 and 6. As I mentioned, many South Africans thought of HIV/AIDS as a modern disease—as a European or American disease that originated abroad. The use of noun classes 5 and 6 was a way to linguistically mark terms for HIV/AIDS as foreign. This particular grammatical feature was important for HIV stigma because it reinforced or even constituted the idea that HIV/AIDS was somehow Other (with a capital O). By using these noun classes, speakers linguistically marginalized those who were infected with HIV. This reflected, and in some cases may have even motivated, various kinds of physical violence, social ostracism, and exclusion.

Marking through Click Consonants

A second linguistic pattern of markedness that may have played a role in the constitution of stigma was the use of click consonants in the standard isiZulu translation of AIDS and a select few other terms. While the links are not immediately evident, I suggest that this appearance of click consonants in the word for AIDS is connected to a historical linguistic patterning of *hlonipha* respect. Historically, *hlonipha* was not only a general moral/ethical ethos of respect avoidance, but also a formalized register of linguistic avoidance (see Agha 1998 on registers of honorific language). In 2008, most South Africans did not use or know about this register. In fact, some university students described reading about it as being like reading about a foreign culture (Finlayson 2002). That archaic avoidance register had relied heavily on click consonants. Historical linguistics suggests that those click consonants became a part of standard isiZulu through incorporation into the *hlonipha* register from other southern African languages (Herbert 1990b).

The historical process of linguistic incorporation relied on the role that click sounds played in marking the foreign (Herbert 1990a; Irvine 1998). Researchers have reconstructed the incorporation of click consonants into the isiZulu lexicon using historical linguistics methods, colonial records, and archaeological evidence. The *hlonipha* avoidance register was related to Zulu kinship and residence patterns that were patrilineal and patrilocal (Vilakazi 1962). Prototypically, when a new bride entered her husband's family's homestead or *kraal*, she was expected to treat elders, especially her father-in-law, deferentially (Doke 1930 [1927]: 378). Transposed into English, that *hlonipha* avoidance register has been explained as follows:

> One could consider the following situation: Robert and Grace Green have three
> children—William, Joan, and Margaret. William marries Mary and takes her

home to his family. Here she is taught a new vocabulary by Joan, her sister-in-law and where necessary advised by Grace, her mother-in-law. This is because from now on she may never use the syllables occurring in the names of her husband's family, i.e. simplistically *rob, ert, green, will, may* and *grace*. Thus for the sentence "Grace will not eat green yoghurt," Mary would have to say something like: "The older daughter of Smith refuses to eat grass-coloured yomix." This (in simplified form) demonstrates the linguistic constraints to which one would be subjected in conforming with this linguistic custom. (Finlayson 2002: 279)

In this hypothetical example, Mary, a new bride, moves from her home to her husband's family's home (patrilocal residence) and must learn a new vocabulary based on the specifics of family names to signal respect to her new family who will be elders and eventually ancestors in her children's lineage (patrilineal descent). A key aspect of indexing respect in this archaic pattern of linguistic reference was the practice of avoiding the syllables of the names of superordinate individuals.

Click consonants became an integral part of Zulu and other *Nguni* languages of southern Africa in the 1700s and 1800s through their use in this *hlonipha* respect register. At that time, click consonants were not found in isiZulu but were part of neighboring Khoi San hunter-gatherer languages. The generally accepted archaeology of the region is that proto-Nguni-speaking agriculturalists migrated to southern Africa over one thousand years ago. This migration initiated an extended period of linguistic and cultural contact with the Khoi San hunter-gatherers who were already occupying the region. Since clicks were not a part of *Nguni* languages, the substitution of click consonants for isiZulu consonants was a relatively simple solution to the problem of linguistic avoidance described in the foregoing yogurt example. By using clicks in the place of other consonants, women performing *hlonipha* were sure to properly avoid pronouncing the syllables of their in-laws' names. By the time European missionaries and scholars were establishing orthographic conventions for isiZulu, click sounds had been incorporated into the language, and the sounds were given their own letters: "c" is used to represent a dental click /|/, "q" a palato-alveolar click /ǂ/,[3] and "x" a lateral click /‖/—each of these may be radical (e.g., "c" /|/), aspirated (e.g., "ch" /|ʰ/), voiced (e.g., "gc," /g|/), or nasal (e.g., "nc" /n|/) (Dent and Nyembezi 1969: vii–viii).

Linguistic anthropologist Judith Irvine (1998) indicates that this daughter-in-law/father-in-law relationship was not the only social space where *hlonipha* was prescribed. Rather, the idea of the daughter-in-law who dutifully performs *hlonipha* toward her father-in-law became a central cultural image linked to a language ideology of social differentiation. Clicks, associated with Khoi San languages, became "*icons* of 'foreignness'" that were projected onto other levels of social organization (Irvine and Gal 2000: 45–46). Such an ideology ignored the ambiguity of the place of Khoi San speakers in Zulu communities, where Khoi San intermarried with Zulu and where there was a hierarchical system of economic co-dependency. In other words, Khoi San individuals lived at the margins of society, but language ideologies of the time erased the ambiguity of their situation and marked Khoi San clicks as an icon of foreignness.

The particular patterning of the click consonant usage in the word most often translated as HIV, *ingculazi*, suggests that click consonants may have retained—at least in this context—some of their earlier ideological significance for marking the foreign. I argue that this was similar to the place of people with HIV/AIDS in many contemporary South African communities—not true outsiders but marked as such through linguistic and communicative practices. Furthermore, this social positioning may have been indicated through the use of clicks for terms for HIV, such as *iqhoks* (high heels), *uqedisizwe* (finisher of the nation), and *ingculazi* (AIDS). Here I briefly focus on the term *ingculazi*, the term often used in isiZulu language translations of medical pamphlets and other information about HIV/AIDS. Though the origins of the word *ingculazi* are unclear, I suggest that the word follows common isiZulu derivational patterns for changing a verb into a noun and for substituting a click consonant for a pulmonic one. The term may in fact be derivative of the isiZulu verb for being sick, *ukugula*. To transform *ukugula* to *ingculazi*, a series of three grammatical shifts must occur (see figure 6.6). The prefix *uku-* (noun class 15, the infinitive verb form) is replaced by noun class nine, which sometimes is used to indicate "the instrument of the action signified by the verb" (Doke 1930 [1927]: 67). In other words, this nominalization of the verb "to be sick" may indicate the entity or thing causing the sickness (part 1 in figure 6.6). A suffix, *azi* (an augmentative suffix), is also added to—*gula* (part 2). Finally, a dental click is added to the voiced velar plosive /g/ (part 3).[4] The use of the dental click here is consistent with historical evidence suggesting that the dental click was the preferred substitute for a pulmonic consonant (Herbert 1990a: 130).

In this analysis, the most literal translation of *ingculazi* might be, "a/the big illness," which closely matches an often-employed English avoidance term

```
(1) uku-   gula   →   in-    gula
    INF-   sick        nc9-   sick
(2) gula          →   gul-   azi
    sick              sick-  AUG
(3) gula          →   gcula
    sick              sick (respect/ avoidance)
```

FIGURE 6.6. Transforming *Ukugula* into *Ingculazi*.

for HIV/AIDS, "the big thing" (Squire 2007). I speculate that the invention of the term *ingculazi* may have occurred within a framework of *hlonipha* avoidance. If this were the case, then click consonants, utilized in the *hlonipha* register through at least the middle of the twentieth century, may have retained at least some vague value as a part of the language of avoidance in 2008. Regardless of the etymology of the term *ingculazi* or the contemporary indexical valences of click consonants, the history of click consonants in Zulu detailed here indicates a long history of ambivalence toward involvement with foreign communities and their languages, as well as a parallel case of utilizing linguistic borrowing in order to mark a class of people as outsiders. Both cases indicate the centrality of linguistic practices in creating and maintaining ideologies of exclusion.

CONCLUSION

Stigmatizing reference to HIV marked the virus and infected individuals as foreign, Othering people with HIV in ways that allowed for aversion, fears of pollution, and taboo. The language of HIV support utilized by Thembeka choir members and other patient-activists, described throughout this book, was a creative transformation of these language ideologies associated with the linguistic markedness of HIV stigma. Supportive reference to HIV likewise marked the virus as foreign and indexically linked infected individuals with the foreign, but this was a powerful entity that was ideologically positioned as foreign, namely biomedicine/global health. These kinds of reference to HIV were closely linked to the transposition of HIV discussed in the previous chapter. Choir members transposed biomedical models of not only HIV/AIDS but also understandings of disclosure and responsibility (more on this in chapter 7). Both stigma and support were constituted at the borders of linguistic and cultural systems, rooted in the play between English and isiZulu, between Zulu spiritual traditions and biomedicine.

More generally, the foregoing discussion demonstrates how literature on language ideologies and markedness both informs and could respond to anthropological scholarship on stigma. This provides the basis for a theorization of the role of language—in particular language ideologies and sociolinguistic markedness—in the constitution of stigma, as well as an examination of how the linguistic constraints of markedness and language ideologies shape creative responses to stigma. The choir's existence as a bio-speech community, as well as their verbal repertoire that included the transposition of HIV across contexts in activities of narrating, joking about, and singing about HIV, was meaningful in part in response to these linguistic patterns of stigmatization and the linguistic constraints of isiZulu and English.

Finally, this chapter's analysis of the linguistic patterns of stigma and support also indicates that discussions of exclusion and stigma should include contemporary models of globalization, global circulation, and, more generally, the porous boundaries of communities and societies. Marginalized or excluded people may find social space for support by making connections with groups or individuals conceptualized as outsiders (see also Besnier 2011). The choir's creative responses to HIV emerged from cultural contact with South African doctors, American researchers, and international aid workers. By turning a language ideology of exclusion on its head, group members were able to transform the linguistic marking of HIV into an indication of the choir's exceptionalism. In particular, musical, humorous, and narrative performance provided group members with the limited ability to traverse semiporous boundaries of global health groups, to connect to doctors, researchers, and aid workers who acted as gatekeepers to money, medication, and other resources of the global AIDS assemblage. In a globalized context involving the uneven circulation of resources, discourses, and entities across communities of speakers, the Thembeka choir creatively transposed HIV/ AIDS and in the process transformed stigma into support and activism.

7 · PERFORMANCE AND THE TRANSPOSITION OF A GLOBAL HEALTH ETHICS OF DISCLOSURE

"There's a certain sense of shame. Activism helps people expunge that. Your identity can never be reduced to three letters of the alphabet or to a disease. But the minute you assume your HIV status as something that is part of your life, not something to be proud or ashamed of, but something you live with, the prejudice and the stigma become someone else's problem."

—Antiapartheid and AIDS Activist Zackie Achmat

In May 2013, I return to Durban to do follow-up fieldwork, and I am invited to a *braai* at Bongiwe's (as mentioned earlier in the book). After Amahle and I have stopped to visit her boyfriend, we pick up Thulani and Siphesihle and we drive back across town, up a very long and winding hill, past some taxi ranks that are marred by frequent shootings, and into an informal settlement area. Bongiwe has arranged for me to lock my rental car at her neighbor's home just down the hill. It is still a difficult drive up a steep, wet, very bumpy set of wheel ruts through areas full of greenery. Then it is a short walk up a footpath to her home. Bongiwe and her husband, who passed away in 2012, had paid for this house to be built with hard-earned money (discussed earlier in the book). After many renovations, her house is now quite comfortable—much like township homes—with several rooms, a flush toilet, running water, cinder block walls, and a corrugated iron roof. Soon after we arrive, we light the coals and start cooking meat, looking out over the verdant valley sparsely populated with self-made homes. I stand outside with the men at the grill, while the women work inside to prepare salads and side dishes. Everyone is happy to see each other, and we spend most of the time joking with one another.

After we finish cooking and grilling, the men and women meet inside in Bongiwe's family room and squeeze onto three comfortable couches. Everyone is taking pictures of each other with their cell phones as they eat, mouths full of marinated meat. Siphesihle playfully performs a caricature of stuffing himself silly. As people start to settle down, Thulani stands up to make an announcement. He starts with a prayer, thanking God for the meal, the company, and my visit. Then he tells everyone that I have something I want to talk about. I previously told him my plans about writing a book and my desire to discuss these plans with the choir. Though choir members had technically provided informed consent for this in 2008, in ethical practice consent is best thought of as an ongoing process. At this time, I feel the need to discuss the book project with group members. I take the floor, explaining that I am hoping to gain approval from the choir to write and publish a book based on my research experiences. I say that I will work to make sure that the group would be compensated if I were to make any money from sales of the book.

"No, Steve, don't worry about the money," Siphesihle interjects. "If it comes then it comes. We're not worried about that now." This is a nice sentiment and an expression of his trust in me, especially in the context of the group's ongoing internal struggles about whether they are being exploited and whether some choir members are monopolizing resources of doctors and aid organizations. I continue to explain the book, passing around a recently published ethnography about an Indian township in Durban as an example.

I finish with what I consider to be a side note, assuring the group, "Of course, I will use pseudonyms and everyone will remain anonymous." In my mind, this is a given and is ancillary to the main issue of whether or not the book idea will be approved.

A brief silence fills the room.

Then, a chorus of voices reply one after another, "I don't have a problem if you use my real name," and "yes, it's fine if you use our real names."

I am surprised that this is what group members are focusing on, after the lengthy explanation of the book project—though in retrospect I realize that it makes sense. Many people in this group have become HIV counselors. They have gained economic and social capital through revealing their HIV-positive status to others, using disclosure as a form of support and activism. Indeed, disclosure—the term used by research participants in English and isiZulu—is highly valued among members of the choir.

I am uncertain as to how to respond. Should I rewrite my study documents that detailed all the steps I would take to protect research participants' real identities? Would the institutional review board at Georgia State University even accept this as the choir's wish? So much of my project has been built around the problems presented by stigma and my desire to learn more about facing stigma without revealing research participants' identities.

After a minute or so of vocal assertions that it would be okay to use people's real names, Siphesihle's brother (who, as mentioned, is also HIV positive and who attended many choir rehearsals) speaks up. He reminds choir members that even though they might be okay with revealing their HIV status to others, they could have family members or future partners, spouses, or children who might prefer anonymity. Here, I think he is speaking not only for himself but also for nonpresent (and imagined future) kin, spouses, partners, and children. Eventually, choir members agree that I should maintain anonymity.

This discussion about anonymity versus disclosure showcases two alternative, sometimes conflicting, moral/ethical discourses about HIV disclosure that were prevalent in South Africa (Seidel 1993). The first discourse, which circulated alongside the resources, medication, and people of international aid, emphasized that individuals had a responsibility to disclose. In this discourse, HIV disclosure was a way to increase awareness of HIV and make sure that the disease did not spread through unprotected sexual contact with partners who did not know of one's positive status. This meant that access to resources was tied, in part, to the ability to perform disclosure (to international audiences, at least). The second discourse, which was tied to South African ideals about *hlonipha* (respect) introduced earlier in the book, emphasized that one had a responsibility to a wide web of social relationships, especially kin relationships, and thus should often *not* disclose out of respect for those social relationships. This discourse sometimes reinforced HIV stigma. It did not necessarily prohibit disclosure, but it did highly limit it.

Moral/ethical discourses may shape actions by providing guidance for how one should or could act in the course of everyday encounters. In reality, though, much of what comes to be thought of as moral/ethical is first enacted in the unplanned temporal unfolding of everyday life (García 2014; Zigon

2009). Significant experiential distinctions can be made between everyday habitual (communicative) acts, on the one hand, and conscious (often linguistically articulated) reflection on what one should or could do, on the other hand. The former is sometimes labeled "moral," while the latter is sometimes labeled "ethical" (Foucault 1993; Robbins 2009: 278). I tend to use the combined terms "moral/ethical" and "morality/ethics." This usage represents a theoretical stance that is compatible with linguistic anthropology (see Zigon and Throop 2014: fn. 1). As mentioned in earlier discussions of reflexivity, communicative actions are significant in the production of intermediate, not fully coherent experiences of reflection (Throop 2003: 235). In the case of actual human encounters, it is not evident that a researcher should often be able to decide whether or not a person's experience is reflexive enough to be categorized as ethical rather than moral. For this reason, and because linguistic anthropology locates morality/ethics first and foremost in communicative encounters (Rumsey 2010), I use the combined term "morality/ethics."

This chapter examines two moral/ethical discourses that shaped the navigation of disclosure among members of the Thembeka choir and others living with HIV in South Africa. In the chapter, I focus on the role of performance in the navigation of moments of overlap and conflict. Here, morality/ethics is part and parcel of—and a response to—stigmatization (Kleinman 2006; Yang et al. 2007). Stigmatized individuals often have a "moral career" or moral trajectory (Goffman 1963). Stigma circumscribes the activities that marked individuals should or could engage in, and often, marked individuals respond by creating or immersing themselves in alternative moral/ethical discourses that help them to face stigma in everyday life. One key aspect of anthropological analysis of such topics is the contact, overlap, and conflict between multiple cultural understandings of morality/ethics (e.g., Robbins 2007; Zigon 2009); another is the ways that morality/ethics is encoded in linguistic patterns and constituted through communicative practices (e.g., Duranti 1994; Keane 2011; Lambek 2010). This chapter examines the role of performance, in everyday life and on stage, in the choir's ability to transpose a moral/ethical stance on HIV disclosure associated with global health into contexts that included home community audiences.

The Thembeka choir's simultaneous engagement with the two moral/ethical discourses discussed here was a key part of their connections to the multiple, overlapping social networks of global health and South African life: international aid groups, funding agencies, American researchers and doctors, South African doctors and global health professionals, and Durban-area neighbors and family. In general, Americans, Europeans, and those closely associated with biomedicine and global health tended to embrace the moral/ethical discourse of individual rights and responsibilities, while neighbors, family, and other black South African support group members tended to embrace the moral/ethical discourse of duties and respect in social/ familial context. Thembeka choir members, in particular, were sometimes able to leverage the unique communicative properties of performance to transpose a global health moral/ethical discourse into home community contexts and thus satisfy the requirements of both moral/ethical frameworks.

DISCLOSURE AS PROCESS AND PERFORMANCE

As mentioned in the previous chapter, disclosure is most often an ongoing process rather than a single communicative act (Clemente Pesudo 2005; Liang 1997). Disclosure is not only a process but also a performance—not in the sense of being insincere, but rather in the sense of being a communicative process that shares properties in common with other instances of performance. This understanding of disclosure is useful for understanding how group members dealt with the ambiguity of negotiating the two overlapping moral/ethical discourses of HIV disclosure. In fact, in some cases performance allowed choir members to satisfy the requirements of both moral/ ethical discourses at the same time. This was the case at a kids' soccer match organized by one choir member, Sthembile.

Sthembile, a choir member in her thirties with two young children, was very involved with sports. She had played sports as an adolescent, and she volunteered as a coach for her daughter's netball[1] team and her son's soccer team. She lived in an informal settlement not far from where I rented an apartment, just over the hill from the prestigious University of KwaZulu-Natal campus. Her house was tiny—probably less than 400 square feet—but well made. It included one bedroom, a very small living area and attached kitchen, and a small bathroom. There were always kids around her house. Sthembile had taken it upon herself to be an informal mentor and, as part of her mentoring activities, to be an informal HIV activist. She thought it would be fun to organize a soccer match between the choir and one of the boys' teams, ages 12 and under. Of course, we would also have to host a *braai*.

It is early September 2008. The choir decides to have the soccer match at a park not too far from the Durban Hospital clinic and very close to a popular local mall. The park is in a predominantly middle-class neighborhood, which means that it is well maintained. It consists of a large rectangle of trimmed grass bisected by a paved path and some shrubbery. A soccer field covers most of the north side. Once again, I find myself traveling to a nearby place where Amahle knows she can purchase quality meat at a low price, loading up the car and making our way over to the playing field. Sthembile has borrowed some red jerseys from an older boys' team. The younger boys' team show up in their blue and yellow jerseys. I had played soccer as a kid, specializing as a goalkeeper, so I volunteer for that position. I am way too tall for the goalkeeper shorts that are provided. We all think that I look pretty funny in them! As the boys' team warms up, we stand around in our jerseys joking with one another about how we shouldn't go too easy on the other team. They look diminutive, but we are old, after all. The game begins. The boys demolish us. It is not even a contest. Siphesihle's brother is playing, but without proper sports shoes. One of his loafers breaks about ten minutes into the match. He keeps playing, hobbling around the field and smiling. After the boys have finished teaching us a lesson about soccer, we retire to the side of the field for our *braai*. Everyone has had a great time. I let Zethu's son play with the camera and film some of the meal. We clean up and everyone goes home.

Not once during the soccer match does anyone mention anything about HIV. Still, Sthembile considers our match to be an example of AIDS activism. The boys on the soccer team know that the choir is an HIV support group, and Sthembile has spoken with various children about HIV at different moments in the past. To her, the important thing is that the boys have seen that this group of people living with HIV is cool, happy, and healthy. Through the soccer match they have learned a lesson—that not all people with HIV look sick and skinny. Sthembile thinks that this might cause the boys to think twice rather than assuming that any healthy-looking sexual partner is uninfected.

This soccer match event is a good example of the idea that disclosure is often an ongoing process rather than a single communicative act. It does not always take the form of one person sitting down with another and saying, "I am HIV positive." Disclosure might mean first letting someone know that you go to the hospital regularly, then taking one's ARVs in front of that person or displaying some sort of knowledge about the scientific model of the virus. There may be social activities in which some participants know a person's HIV-positive status while others do not. And it may take several conversations to get to a point of verbal disclosure. For the choir and the boys' soccer team, disclosure meant playing sports and eating a meal together after Sthembile had a conversation with the boys about the choir.

TWO MORAL/ETHICAL DISCOURSES: RIGHTS VERSUS DUTIES

During the *braai* described at the beginning of the chapter, when choir members articulated their acceptance of the use of their real names, they were enacting one of the two prominent moral/ethical discourses about HIV disclosure. This discourse, associated with biomedicine and global health, is linked to neoliberalism but can be traced in Eurasia back to Hellenic philosophy of the fourth century B.C.E. (Aristotle 1998 [4th century B.C.E.]). The moral/ethical discourse of rights and responsibilities emphasizes the individually centered nature of morality/ethics (what rights and responsibilities does an individual have?). While scholars from Nietzsche (1966 [1907]) to Foucault (1986) have critiqued and deconstructed this understanding of morals/ethics, it remains dominant in many Christian teachings. Choir members and other South Africans would have been exposed to this moral/ethical philosophy from a young age when they began attending churches of various denominations. Historically, as mentioned, Christianity has been dominant throughout much of the country for over one hundred years (Elphick and Davenport 1997). Though the moral/ethical discourse of rights and responsibilities was, at one point, a European import, it is now part of the cultural fabric of South African society.

AIDS activism in South Africa was globally situated. Responses to AIDS stigma were tied to the Judeo-Christian moral underpinnings of the embodied habitual standpoints of global health professionals and activists. Such understandings of the morality/ethics of disclosure were similar to other neoliberally influenced discourses of disclosure (e.g., in some LGBT activism) where disclosure was equated with progressive activism while nondisclosure was linked to stigma and denial (Duggan 2002; Zigon 2011). These standpoints were reinforced by and expanded on in the Christian-influenced priorities and policies of funding agencies, such as George W. Bush's creation of PEPFAR. For instance, the first two letters of the "ABCs" of public health prevention—abstain and be faithful—attest to this, and for years much aid funding was tied to an explicit rejection of activism that included safe sex messaging. More broadly, as activists, choir members tended to adopt the Christian/Hellenic virtue-oriented discourse that was the basis of many global health interventions.

The Benefits of Knowledge (the Moral/Ethical Discourse of Rights)

As mentioned in chapter 3, during fieldwork I asked Amahle to interview some of her friends and former choir members living with HIV in isiZulu (e.g., figure 3.2). The interviews she (and I) conducted were not intended to be representative of interviewees' inner lives or selves. Rather, they became "sites for the discursive construction of identity" (Bucholtz 2011: 38). As discussed in previous chapters, an AIDS activist identity was evident in many of these interviews. One woman that Amahle interviewed, named Rachel, had been a member of the choir and support group years before I arrived in South Africa. Like Amahle and like most of the other choir members, Rachel was an isiZulu-speaking black South African in her mid-thirties who lived in one of the neighborhoods surrounding Durban. When Amahle interviewed Rachel, the two spoke at length about the benefits of "knowledge." This discussion foregrounded the moral/ethical discourse of rights and responsibilities that was associated with neoliberalism and Christian virtue ethics.

It is September 2008. Amahle has invited Rachel to her township home to conduct an interview in privacy. I am also present. Even if I had been absent, though, I would have been an imagined future audience, because Amahle is recording the interview. At the outset, Rachel explains that when she first fell ill, she knew to get tested for HIV because her cousin had also become very ill and been diagnosed as HIV positive. Amahle then borrows the English verb "to benefit" to ask Rachel about how her cousin's experiences have impacted her own understanding of her illness. Amahle asks (in isiZulu, with English code-mixing indicated in bold), "Did you see that helping you? Did you **benefit** from already knowing that?"

Amahle's question is not ideal from the standpoint of conducting an interview. Amahle's question leads Rachel in a particular direction in two ways. First, Amahle uses verbs like "help" and "benefit" rather than more neutral words such as "impact" or "affect." She assumes, or has previous knowledge, that Rachel is aided by the knowledge of her cousin's HIV status. Second, Amahle borrows the verb "benefit" from English, leading Rachel to respond in kind with English borrowings.

Rachel replies (in isiZulu), "Mhm, it helped me a lot. It helped me a lot. **Because,** I will say, my husband, because we were about to get married, this was where he showed me whether he loved me or not, because when I **disclosed** to him, we separated because I am **HIV positive.**" Here, Amahle's use of the English "benefit" and Rachel's use of "disclose" and "HIV positive" correspond with the pattern discussed throughout the book of utilizing English terms associated with medicine to positively value an association with the foreign and to transpose HIV/AIDS across communicative contexts.

Amahle and Rachel's conversation seemed almost choreographed. It was as if they had read a set of talking points and were sticking to them. The idea that disclosure could benefit others by spreading awareness and knowledge was a part of a much larger discourse—a discourse that was circulating through support groups and activist organizations in South Africa and globally. That discourse was one of individual rights (rights to medication, treatment, and freedom from discrimination) and individual responsibilities (the responsibility to take one's medication regularly—or stick to the "regimen"— and to disclose to others). While it was ultimately oriented toward a larger social good, this discourse was individual centered in the sense that it prescribed individual disclosure regardless of the immediate audience. In other words, disclosure was an action taken by a virtuous *individual* regardless of social context. The general concept of individual responsibility (to disclose) was linked to ideals of the individual as the bearer of inalienable rights and to the Eurasian tradition of virtue ethics introduced earlier. Furthermore, these concepts were connected to neoliberal approaches to care that relied on individuals rather than governments to perform care-oriented actions, neoliberal approaches that have been documented in international aid groups whose (European and American) employees and volunteers may themselves subscribe to such notions (Nguyen 2010; Robins 2008; Zigon 2011). In some cultural contexts, people also conceptualized these notions to be linked to ideals of modernity and linked to the English language (Boellstorff 2009: 352).

Across multiple interviews in my fieldwork, this moral/ethical discourse framed individuals as either disclosers or nondisclosers, as people who "accepted" their status or did not. This discourse focused on issues of acceptance, (sexual) partners, and care. In theory, it was not necessarily linked to tenets of biomedicine, including concepts of CD4 counts, viral loads, and ARVs. However, the two had become entwined into a single moral/ethical discourse, not only in South Africa but in many contexts where development and aid organizations had become involved with the pandemic (Nguyen 2008: 131). In Amahle's interview with Rachel, the two performed this moral/ethical discourse of rights and responsibilities that was oriented especially toward imagined future audiences of researchers, students, and aid organizations (including readers of this book).

A Chorus of *Hlonipha* (the Moral/Ethical Discourse of Respect)

Choir members' ideas about one's individual responsibility to disclose regardless of audience or social context contrasted with my observation of some of choir members' behaviors in everyday life. There, I found that stigma and disclosure were often treated as ongoing and processual, as mentioned. In everyday life, choir members and others living with HIV also drew from another moral/ethical discourse that emphasized a person's duties based on social roles. Whereas Christianity, biomedicine, and global neoliberal capitalism made the moral/ethical discourse of rights and responsibilities a significant force in the AIDS pandemic, notions of home and African tradition centered the moral/ethical discourse of duties and respect in the South African epidemic. Remember that the idea of respect, or *hlonipha*, refers to a set of culturally specific prescriptions for how to indicate respect, and that at one point in time this included a linguistic *hlonipha* register. The underlying moral/ethical logic of this ideal of *hlonipha* is distinct from the moral/ethical logic of virtue. In the Hellenic-Christian tradition, virtue is the purview of the individual. It is a set of principles guiding individual action. While the execution might change based on the social situation, the underlying principles remain the same. With *hlonipha*, on the other hand, what counts as moral or ethical depends on the specifics of different social relationships and the social roles that one holds and the specific social contexts in which one finds oneself. In this discourse, it is not the act of HIV disclosure that is immoral but rather the act of disclosing in circumstances when that disclosure might be injurious to one's parents and other kin. As the next story shows, it was still possible for choir members to disclose to their parents. However, disclosure was supposed to happen in a "respectful" manner.

As mentioned, the Thembeka choir had been the subject of two documentaries. In one of those documentaries, which was directed by American film students, Amahle and Zethu disclosed to their parents. When Amahle described this in her speech to American Fulbright students (discussed in chapter 4), she introduced the story of her disclosure to their parents as follows:

In two thousand and four—two thousand and four? Yes. The Americans . . . there were four of them, they visited here in South Africa. They wanted to meet the choir. They wanted to meet us because they [had] already heard about us while we were in the U.S. They came to see us. They did a documentary. They said anyone who wants to talk about HIV/AIDS can come and talk and give his or her evidence [about] being HIV positive.

[At] that time it was not easy for me to talk about HIV though. I'm [being] upset that I'm HIV positive. I can tell everybody that through music, but not just standing in front of everybody and telling them, no, I'm HIV positive, duh duh duh, all those things. Then I said no, it's not easy for me to just talk about it because it makes me cry maybe if I'm just talking about it.

Then one day my sister, [she] was one of those who were doing the documentary, they came home and they did the documentary at [our] home. On the following day, I asked my sister, okay you can give me this telephone number for these people so that I can call them.

When Amahle met with the documentary film students they asked her about her family—where were her parents living? What was it like living on the farm? Open and generous as always, Amahle invited the filmmakers to visit her parents on the farm. This led the filmmakers to ask if her parents knew her status. Amahle replied that Zethu was not ready to disclose because of concerns about their mother's health. Their mother had suffered a stroke, and they were worried about the impact that disclosure might have on her.

Zethu and Amahle eventually decided that they could disclose to their parents with the help of the choir. They made a plan. The group and the filmmakers drove out to the rural area where the sisters' parents lived, vehicles loaded with not only camera equipment and choir members but also enough food and supplies to have a nice party. The ostensible purpose of their visit was to show the filmmakers what the rural area was like. Much of the event was captured in the documentary. Significantly, while the parents did learn about the sisters' HIV status, Zethu and Amahle did not tell their parents directly. Instead, the choir first performed in the family's sitting room. Then, Fanele took the parents into another room. Fanele told them that everyone in the choir was HIV positive. She had been trained as an HIV counselor and used that training to explain some basic facts about HIV to the parents, being careful to emphasize that an HIV-positive diagnosis was not a death sentence. Amahle told me that her father was very sweet after that event. He called regularly to ask how the two sisters were doing, making sure that they were taking care of themselves and going to the doctor when they had any symptoms of illness.

I had heard other stories of disclosure to parents that had gone wrong. Some people had been kicked out of their parents' homes when they revealed that they were HIV positive. What made Amahle and Zethu's situation different? No doubt, an important difference was the people involved and their life histories. Remember that Amahle had been in and out of hospitals for her whole life. Her parents were the ones who had taken her to the doctor. Throughout their lives they had engaged significantly with biomedicine. In this context, an important part of the sisters' reluctance to disclose may simply have been the difficulty of telling their parents that not one but two of their children were infected with a chronic or terminal sexually transmitted disease.

The specific concerns of the sisters and the way they disclosed also fit the moral/ethical discourse of duties and respect that was prevalent in South Africa. As in other situations, choral singing softened the impact of disclosure by creating an imaginary "fourth wall" of performance. As Amahle explained it, at that time it was not easy for her to talk about HIV, but she had fewer issues performing for audiences that knew that everyone in the group was HIV positive. In addition, having the other choir members with her diffused responsibility for the message. In terms of *hlonipha* (respect), perhaps the most important aspect of this event was that it was another unrelated choir member who pulled the parents aside and disclosed for the sisters. In this way, Zethu and Amahle were able to maintain their respectful relationship to their parents while also allowing the parents to learn of their HIV-positive status. They fulfilled their duty as children and displayed *hlonipha* while simultaneously transposing the moral/ethical discourse of individual responsibility to disclose into this family context.

"The Boys Are Negative!"

In contrast with such examples of successful HIV disclosure, there were times when group members faced the limits of their ability to transpose a global health understanding of disclosure into home community contexts. In these instances, distinctions arose between those choir members who had disclosed more widely and those who had not. One significant moment with regard to HIV disclosure and the limits of transposition occurred at the end of the very first rehearsal that I attended and recorded (also discussed in chapter 3). Recall that Siphesihle had not disclosed to his family despite the fact that the choir rehearsed in their garage. At the end of this rehearsal, concerns about how the group would deal with the possible opportunity of appearing on a local documentary TV show led to a critical discussion about disclosure in home communities.

It is March 2008. At the end of choir practice, Thulani calls a group meeting and everyone forms a circle. Thulani begins to speak in hushed tones. I can tell that my video camera's internal microphone is not going to pick up any of the conversation. I am not sure whether I should record or hang back and let people navigate a difficult situation. In this case, I decide to move into the middle of the circle and sit cross-legged with my camera. In doing so, I capture a conversation that would become a central part of my understanding of the choir's complex stance on disclosure and HIV activism.

Thulani begins by telling the group that there is an opportunity to appear on a local TV documentary show hosted by a celebrity named Zola. However, this would require what he calls a "mandate" from the group. After two minutes of explaining some of the details of his thinking, how he got in contact with Zola, and what he thought Zola could do for the group, Thulani says (in isiZulu, English code-mixing in bold) the following:

> Because he has a **studio plus** he has many people who produce him. **So** we often see that he can do things for people, and the things that he does are successful, **but** the thing **will call for disclosure, it will call for** those people to see you, those who see you no matter where they see you there. **And** maybe then you will have to explain where you explain. **But** then it might be an easy way to **accomplish**—or maybe it might be an easy way that we can make a **CD** if we succeed, **so** . . . that is the reason I was saying that I need that **mandate** of that sort.

Here, Thulani has been talking around the subject of disclosure for several minutes and only at this point does he mention it outright. He explains that to appear on this local documentary would be different from previous documentaries and choir performances for international audiences. People from choir members' own neighborhoods would see this documentary. In this sense, working with Zola would be, in and of itself, a disclosure of the HIV-positive status of everyone in the group. While other group activities have allowed individuals to enact the moral/ethical discourse of duties and respect in their homes and neighborhoods, this documentary would be a performance of the moral/ethical discourse of responsibility—responsibility to disclose as a form of activism—in home communities. For this reason, Thulani suggests that he needs approval from the group (a "mandate").

Bongiwe is the first person to respond. She is upset because she thinks that someone has gone behind other group members' backs, talking with Zola, and receiving financial benefits without sharing with the others. Bongiwe's fear about this is part and parcel of the broader concerns mentioned throughout this book that choir members have about fairness in group access to the uneven global circulation of aid. Choir members have repeatedly been worried that one or another group member has unfairly benefited from a friendship with a particular researcher or aid worker and not shared that benefit with others.

Bongiwe is angry, and starts to walk out of the garage, emphasizing (in isiZulu), "Let me go home." Others, including Dumisile, Philani, Siphesihle, Thulani, and Zethu, call Bongiwe back, saying they do not know anything about what she is talking about. After some discussion, Thulani decides that Bongiwe's critique should not affect their current discussion about Zola's documentary. He continues (in isiZulu, English code-mixing in bold): "We, just—the **concern** that we have here—that I have here—are we okay if I say that we do it as a **group**? It will appear, truly, where it appears, and maybe you still have a **problem** . . . that you cannot **address**." Thulani pauses. There is a moment of quiet. What happens next is shown in figure 7.1, with English code-mixing indicated in bold.

In the excerpt in figure 7.1, Zethu incredulously asks Thulani if he is trying to talk about disclosure. Thulani replies, "yeah," prompting one woman to respond, "a long time ago" (line 03). This is followed by Amahle's statement that they have already disclosed. Thulani attempts to put the conversation back on track, working toward a rearticulation of why "this case" might

01	Z:	for *i* disclosure, *uqondise kwi* disclosure?
		For disclosure, are you directing it ((the conversation)) to disclosure?
02	T:	*yah*
		yeah
03	?:	*kade*
		a long time ago
04	A:	*engani sazidisklosa*
		but we have disclosed ((already))
05	T:	*yah, kodwa phela ... noma kwi* this case *seku ukabona //* (???)
		yeah, but truly ... or in this case it is, you see
06	A:	[*(ayifuthi)*
		not again
07		*kuzothiwa amantombazane, abafana ba* negative *abafana amantombazane*
		will it be said that the boys are negative while the girls are
08		a positive. *usholo lokho?*
		positive. Are you talking about that?
09	T:	*sengisholo ukuthi //* in this case-
		I'm saying that in this case
10	C:	[((laughs, slaps thigh))
11	T:	[*(sengisholo ukuthi)*
		I'm saying that
12	D:	[*abafana ba* negative ((smile voice))
		the boys are negative!

FIGURE 7.1. Transcript: The Boys Are Negative (choir rehearsal 3-2-2008, tape 3, 21 min 20 sec). Participants: A = Amahle, C = Celokuhle, D = Dumisile, T = Thulani, Z = Zethu; other participants include Bongiwe, Lethu, Philani, and Siphesihle.

be different, but Amahle interrupts him. She responds in a singsong manner, speeding up the pace of her talk to create a play/joking frame for her talk. She emphasizes that "not again" would it be said that the men of the group are negative while the women are positive.

Months later, when we are transcribing this video together, I ask Amahle about her statement. According to Amahle's annotations, this recalls a time earlier in the choir's history when some neighbors asked men of the choir about the group. Anxious to avoid HIV stigma, the men told these inquiring neighbors that only the women in the choir were HIV positive, that the men were just helping the women with the music out of the goodness of their hearts. This was a betrayal of the support group ideal of sharing and of protecting group members' anonymity.

While this conversation about the local documentary is a serious matter, Amahle voices her concern in a playful manner, goading the men of the group about their previous indiscretion. Twice more, Thulani tries to redirect the conversation back to the topic of the TV documentary (lines 09 and 11), and twice his talk is drowned out by women in the group, first by Celokuhle laughing (line 10) and then by Dumisile's amused comment, "the boys are negative" (line 12). In this excerpt, the implicit acceptance of group members' HIV-positive status is utilized to differentiate women of the choir from the men. The joke is on them (the men) if they think that they are not part of this group of people living with HIV.

After the end of the excerpt in figure 7.1, Thulani persists with his point, explaining again that this would not be like the DVD that was made about them in the past. The women of the group—led by Amahle and Zethu— would have none of this. Amahle then states that they have moved past this issue a long time ago. Zethu adds (in isiZulu), "even if it plays every day like *Generations* we don't have a problem." *Generations* is a South African soap opera that is very popular at this time.

As the conversation continues, it becomes clear that Thulani is concerned about Siphesihle (that he has not disclosed to his family) in particular even though Thulani does not mention him by name. Zethu next insists (shown in figure 7.2) that whoever has a problem "should say so individually." In this way, she and some of the other women single Siphesihle out, goading him to admit that he has not disclosed. Zethu leads the earlier joking to subtly shift into teasing and shaming. By this point in the conversation, the women in the group have fully immersed themselves in their activist personas, adopting a standpoint on disclosure associated with the moral/ ethical discourse of rights and responsibilities. This is done in opposition to the men in the group, after the sore memory of the men's betrayal has resurfaced. Celokuhle insists that if you log on to the Internet you can search for Zethu, find her name along with her HIV-positive status and how long she has been living with the virus (lines 04 and 07). This is an exaggeration. There is information accompanied by some pictures of the choir on the Internet on a website that has not been edited for quite some time, but no individuals' names are listed. When no one responds, Celokuhle singles Siphesihle out, mock-whispering to him, "Why are you so quiet?" (line 10).

01	Z:	oh kay, *ph//ela akasho* individually
		oh kay, truly he/she must say **individually**
02	C:	[(. . . . . . . ???. . . . .) **individually** *uzozake naleyo nkingake*
		(???) individually he/she will come, then, with that problem
03	Z:	*ehheh*
		uh huh
04	C:	**but the rest of the group** *ayikho inkinga uma uloga* **kwi internet** *ufuna*
		but the rest of the group, there is not a problem. If you log into the
		internet looking for
05		uZethu Ngubane
		Zethu Ngubane
06	B?:	*umthole*
		you will find her
07	C:	*uyangena, umthole kuthiwe unengculazi wayithola ngelanga elithize*
		You enter, you will find her, it will say she has AIDS, what day she got it
08		*akusiyona nje imfihlo*
		it's just not a secret
09		((4.0 seconds of silence))
10	C:	((whispering)) *wathula kangaka nje* Siphesihle
		Why are you so quiet Siphesihle?
11	C?:	*ushawa uvalo?*
		Are you scared?
12		((women laughing))
13	S?:	((quietly)) (. . . . . . ???// . . . . .)
14	?:	[*asihambe ma ehke*
		Let's go, then, eh girls?

FIGURE 7.2. Transcript: Are You Scared? (Choir rehearsal 3-2-2008, tape 3, 22 min 30 sec).

She or another woman continue, "Are you scared?" (line 11). One of the men (possibly Siphesihle) attempts to respond, but the women have already stood up to leave.

While men of the choir were able to disclose within the moral/ethical framework of rights and responsibilities in the context of global health encounters (often with non-Zulu interlocutors), they had not been able to do so in the context of encounters with others in their home communities. As discussed, there were times when neither men nor women of the choir disclosed their HIV status. However, in one instance in the past the men of the group had agreed with an assessment that the women were HIV positive but denied the idea that they themselves were HIV positive. This betrayal set the stage for a scathing rebuke by the women. This exchange demonstrated a conflict between the moral/ethical discourse of rights and responsibilities, on the one hand, and the moral/ethical discourse of duties and respect, on the other hand, and revealed a gendered limit in the ability of group members to transpose the moral/ethical discourse associated with HIV activism into their home communities.

PERFORMANCE AND THE EMBODIMENT OF MULTIPLE MORAL/ETHICAL DISCOURSES

Sometimes, Thembeka choir members were able to embody both the moral/ethical discourse of rights and responsibilities and the moral/ethical discourse of duties and respect and thereby transpose a global health orientation toward disclosure into home community contexts. In the example discussed next, the choir was able to perform disclosure and nondisclosure simultaneously to a heterogeneous audience. Analysis of the distinct communicative properties of performance suggest that it was these properties that made such a bivalent embodiment possible. This is an example where performance blurred the boundaries between disclosure and nondisclosure, making it possible to satisfy the demands of both moral/ethical discourses.

Recall that evaluation by an audience, responsibility on the part of performers to that audience, and performers' reflexive attention paid to how they communicate are three key properties of all performances (Bauman and Briggs 1990; Berger and Del Negro 2002). These properties shift the interpretation of communicative actions. When audience members evaluate performers and performers reflexively attend to their speech, both parties begin to search for meaning in the poetics of talk—in the parallel structure of phrases, alliteration, in timing of delivery, in emphasis and prosody. This often makes interpretation more ambiguous (Jakobson 1960). In staged performance, in particular, the co-construction of meaning may become more idiosyncratic as heterogeneous audiences attend to and respond to different aspects of a performance (Bogen 1987). In the example discussed here, these communicative properties of performance allowed the Thembeka choir to simultaneously index disclosure to one audience while indexing *hlonipha* to another.

A Very Positive Wedding

In August 2008, I am invited to attend the wedding of two former choir members, Wendy and Vusi. The bride and groom had been a part of the Thembeka choir, and they had gone on tour to the United States. The couple ask if I would take pictures, videotape the day's events, and create a DVD for them. I think of this as another small way that I can contribute to the lives of research participants (because this means that they will not have to pay for these services). As has become our usual routine, I speak with choir members to arrange transportation. We decide that I will drive to Amahle and Zethu's house, where Thulani and Sthembile will meet us. Then we will go to the wedding together.

I arrive in my rental car at Amahle's house. Sthembile is at the back of the house with Amahle and Zethu, changing out of her kombi clothes (the normal clothes she wore on the minivan taxi ride over to the township) into her nice dress for the wedding. Thulani and I sit on couches in the living room, a space that is by this time very familiar to me from my transcription and interview sessions with Amahle. Thulani starts talking to me about the bride and groom. It is unusual, he explains, for two people with HIV to stick together. There are so many reasons to break up—the psychological trauma of an HIV-positive diagnosis, differing opinions about how to handle stigma and disclosure, and accusations about who is to blame for the infection (had one partner cheated? was this the result of past indiscretion?). In addition to these problems related directly to AIDS, poverty and precarity present financial and social difficulties that lead many South African couples to break up. Wendy and Vusi have persevered—no doubt aided by the fact that Vusi's family is better off financially than many other choir members' families. Everyone at the wedding will be celebrating this wonderful occasion. But, Thulani continues, the choir will have a special reason to celebrate. He also informs me that while the groom's family knows the couple's HIV-positive status, some in the bride's family do not.

After everyone is finished getting ready, we drive to a Catholic church in the township for the official wedding ceremony. The church is tall and cavernous with dark brown bricks. The interior is lined with rows of wooden pews that face an altar at the front of the church. In many ways, the ceremony is like other church weddings I have seen in the United States—happy people decked out in their finest suits and dresses, a bride in a white gown, a religious leader vested by the government with the power to legally wed the couple. But there are a few obvious differences too. First, the entire ceremony is conducted in isiZulu. Second, at appropriate moments when people might have cheered in other contexts, many of the women present ululate.[2] Third, there is a lot more singing than there had been at any wedding I have ever attended previously. And fourth, during the processional and recessional the men and women going down the aisle perform a fun dance step as they walk, adding some flair to the procession.

After the conclusion of the wedding ceremony, we drive through the winding streets of the township to a community center where the bride and groom have organized a luncheon. The building, a large brick structure, consists of a meeting hall with a few steps up to an elevated stage at one end. The floors are linoleum and the walls are painted a dull yellow—sure signs that this structure was built and is maintained by the government. On one side of the room, curtains close off an area of the stage where a buffet lunch has been set up. Occupying most of the floor space are circular tables covered with white tablecloths and surrounded by folding chairs. Just like they had done at the wedding ceremony, the bride, groom, and close family and friends perform a processional dance. This time their walk is accompanied by the thumping bass beat of South African house music blasting from the large speakers that a DJ has set up at the edge of the stage.

After everyone settles in, it is time to get lunch from the buffet. The food is similar to what I have eaten at *braai* after *braai*—grilled beef, chicken, and pork; stiff *paap* (a cornmeal dish similar to polenta or grits); a salad of lettuce, tomatoes, and onions; and spicy beans. We sit down to eat. The choir has chosen a table at the back of the hall and are sitting together, getting a little raucous, having a great time, and using their cell phones and my camera to take many pictures of each other eating the tasty food.

Then it is time for the speeches. The choir is invited up to the stage to formally open the luncheon with a few songs, beginning with a musical version of the prayer, "Our Father Who Art in Heaven" (an arrangement by the choir). Before they perform, though, Thulani takes the microphone and performs a short speech.

"*Sanibonani bakithi* (hello my people)," he begins.

"*Yebo* (hello[3])" replies the audience, sitting at their lunch tables.

Thulani: *Nje ukuhighlighta noma ukuthinta izinto ezithize ngaleli* **choir**. *Umuntu obekade ebona* u**Wendy** *uma edonsa izikhwama ethi uya phesheya ehamba naleli* **choir**. *Uma ethi uya e***Melika** u**Wendy** *ubehamba naleli* **choir**, *uma ethi uya e***London** u**Wendy** *ubehamba naleli* **choir**. *So, i* **choir** *leli nje noma lingaphelele kumanje,* **it's one of those** *abasebenze umsebenzi omkhulu kakhulu ezingeni lokucula.*

English translation

Thulani: But just to **highlight** or to point out some things about this **choir**. A person who was seeing **Wendy**, if she was pulling bags, she was saying she was going overseas, she was going with this **choir**. If she was saying she was going to **America**, **Wendy** was going with this **choir**. If she was saying she was going to **London**, **Wendy** was going with this **choir**. So, this **choir**, just, while it isn't all here now, **it's one of those,** that did very good work with its singing.

FIGURE 7.3. Transcript: Performing Two Discourses of Disclosure (performance 8-2-2008, tape 3, 11 min 35 sec).

Thulani exclaims, "*Sanibonani bo!* (I said hello!)," prompting the people eating their lunches to repeat with more gusto, "*Yebo!*" This classic method of repetition and exclamation, used to get people's attention and solidify their role as an audience, is one way that Thulani frames his talk as performance. In addition, he is standing on a stage and holding a microphone. By repeating his greeting and expecting a unified response, Thulani creates an audience out of the various tables of people sitting, eating, and talking.

Thulani continues with a disclaimer of performance. Though it might seem counterintuitive, in many performance contexts, a disclaimer is a way of framing one's talk as performance through the downplaying of one's virtuosity (which thus draws attention to it) (Bauman 1975). Thulani explains (in isiZulu), "All right, all right, this is nothing special people." He continues (shown in figure 7.3 as spoken [on the left] and in translation [on the right], with code-mixing indicated in bold). What, exactly, did Thulani mean when he said that the choir did very good work with its singing? Why did he spend so much time talking about going abroad? And why did he switch into English, saying "it's one of *those*," with an emphasis on "those"?

In my analysis, Thulani's speech was well crafted to speak to his heterogeneous audience that could be distinguished according to two overlapping divisions: first, those who knew the choir's role as an HIV support and AIDS activist group versus those who did not; and second, those who understood

If... she was saying she was going overseas, she was going with this choir.
[... ...FRAME... ... ...] FOCUS [... ...FRAME... ... ...]

If she was saying she was going to America, Wendy was going with this choir.
[... ...FRAME... ... ...] FOCUS [... ...FRAME... ... ...]

If she was saying she was going to London, Wendy was going with this choir.
[... ...FRAME... ... ...] FOCUS [... ...FRAME... ... ...]

FIGURE 7.4. Parallelism in Action.

disclosure primarily through the moral discourse of rights and responsibilities versus those who understood disclosure primarily through the moral discourse of duties and respect. Thulani included a heavy dose of parallelism in
his speech. "Parallelism" refers to the process wherein a verbal artist repeats
a particular grammatical structure but inserts a new term or phrase into that
structure. It has been suggested that parallelism is the core defining feature
of poetics (Jakobson 1960). One way to theorize parallelism is to identify
part of a phrase as the "frame" (the part that stays the same) and part as the
"focus" (the part that changes). Figure 7.4 provides an analysis of the parallelism of Thulani's speech (in English translation).

Through parallel grammatical constructions, Thulani established the idea
that the choir was a group that had repeatedly gone on tour. While anyone
hearing this could take from it that the choir was a successful group, people
who knew that the choir was an AIDS activist organization could also interpret it as a statement of the value of the group's outreach efforts.

Thulani also made that emphatic switch into English to say, "it's one of
those." Most of his English usage in the speech was conventional and widely
used: choir, *eMelika* (to America), and *eLondon* (to London). After his only
other nonconventional use of English, *ukuhighlighta* (to highlight), Thulani
immediately switched into isiZulu to repeat himself. This suggests to me that
he may have been making a concerted effort to speak primarily in isiZulu
(often his talk was peppered with English words in everyday conversations).
Speaking in isiZulu may have been an accommodation to the parents and
other older people in the audience, some of whom did not speak much
English. In this communicative and social context, Thulani's switch into
English strongly emphasizes his next statement. Indeed, across cultural con-

texts, code-mixing or code-switching for emphasis has been identified as a key facet of multilingual conversation (Gumperz 1982). The choir had not simply done good work with its singing. It was **one of those** types of choir that had done very good work. The switch into English may have also provided an indexical link to the transposition of biomedical models of HIV/AIDS for people familiar with the choir.

By using these poetic and communicative devices within a performance frame, Thulani was able to index the choir's activist work without explicitly disclosing. He was able to point toward the choir's role as an HIV support group and AIDS activist organization, positively valuing that work, without discussing HIV/AIDS outright. At the same time, he provided the choir's standard cover story, namely that they were simply a performance troupe. Before the group began to sing the "Our Father" prayer, Thulani concluded his speech by inviting people to come talk to him and the others, saying (in isiZulu), "Eh, I can't say [much] then [about] this choir. I want you to come close to us when we are eating and find out who this choir is," and then laughing. This was, perhaps, a subtle way of suggesting that a wedding where some family members did not know the bride and groom's status was not a place where he could disclose publicly.

PERFORMANCE AND TRANSPOSITION

The communicative properties of performance made it possible for Thulani to ambivalently point toward both of the moral/ethical discourses about disclosure discussed earlier. Thulani was responsible to the audience (and evaluated by them) for both the form and the content of his words. Though it is difficult to determine whether or not Thulani's cognitive attention was directed toward increased reflexivity, his linguistic reflexivity was clear. After saying hello, he began with a metapragmatic assessment (a bit of talk about the pragmatic force and function of his speech), explaining, "just to highlight or to point out some things about this choir." Here, Thulani was attending to his own talk, characterizing the rest of his speech as accomplishing the social action of "highlighting" or "pointing out" things about the choir. Increased awareness of and attention to communication itself meant that audience members looked beyond the referential content of Thulani's words to interpret his meaning. He emphasized, "it's one of *those* [choirs] that did very good work," allowing members of a heterogeneous audience to interpret the phrase in multiple ways.

More generally, the examples discussed in this chapter demonstrate how Thembeka choir members navigated two overlapping, but sometimes conflicting, moral/ethical discourses—one rooted in notions of individual virtue and the other rooted in notions of social embeddedness and respect. These two overlapping discourses were linked to the multiple audiences to which this choir bio-speech community was oriented on stage and in everyday life: American researchers, doctors, aid workers, donors, global health professionals, South African doctors, other support group members, patient-activists, neighbors, family, and friends. Performance made it possible to sometimes transpose a global health moral/ethical discourse about disclosure into a social context where a Zulu moral/ethical discourse of respect was the default.

8 · CONCLUSION

It is August 2008, and I am at the evening party and ceremony for Wendy and Vusi's wedding celebration (discussed in chapter 7). This part of the party is held at Vusi's family home, which is located near Umlazi township. The night's events include traditional Zulu dancing and singing (*ukusina*), a display of gift-giving in which the bride's family demonstratively covers the groom's family in blankets and gives them other home goods, and a feast of meat sacrificed for the occasion. When it is time to eat, men are directed toward one large tent erected in the backyard and women are directed to another. However, choir members and I eat together on the side of the house, sharing a large platter of meat. It is dark, the space between the house and a retaining wall is relatively narrow, and there is no place to sit. Siphesihle and Thulani take turns playfully taking up the role of server. They hold the platter and offer it to others. I am not able to subtly ask for an explanation as to why we are eating separately, and I do not want to ask explicitly due to my worries about the possibility of disclosure to overhearers. I wonder, is it because I am with them? Because they are known by some to be HIV positive? Or simply because they want to eat together as a group?

While we are eating, I speak to Thulani about an idea he and the others have been discussing for a choir retreat (briefly discussed in chapter 4). Group members want to have a retreat to discuss the direction the group is taking. Trying to be helpful and avoid excessive costs associated with renting a conference room or other space for a retreat, I suggest that the choir could have its retreat at my apartment. Thulani says no, that they need to be far away from everything to clear their minds.

Throughout the month of August, group members continue to think about a retreat. When I speak to Amahle about it, she recounts an exchange she has had with Philani: Philani told her they need a retreat; she replied that she did not have money. Philani suggested that she must organize a way to save for the retreat, and she retorted that she did not have money to spend "on nothing." Amahle thinks that the retreat would be a waste of money and that the choir could just as easily meet all day in the garage where they normally rehearse. The distinction between Amahle's and Thulani's perspectives—that they could hold a discussion anywhere, on the one hand, or that they needed to go far away to have privacy and isolation, on the other hand—is an indication of rifts that are developing within the group.

By September, the choir has decided to hold the retreat. One day, I drive Philani onto the dirt roads near a forest outside of the city of Pietermaritz-burg to check out a place where his friend works that specializes in corpo-rate retreats. The next day, I meet with Philani, Amahle, Siphesihle, Zethu, and Sthembile at Gugu Dlamini Park in downtown Durban (a picture of the park is provided in figure 6.1). Philani shares a packet of information that talks about the retreat location and the various sorts of team-building exercises that are part of the retreat. Everyone decides that we will bring our own food and cook to save money, and I offer to rent a kombi to transport everyone to the retreat. The choir members also come up with general rules that Siphe-sihle playfully reads off to us: no kids, no late-comers, do your hairstyles at your own risk and no accessories such as earrings (which is a joking way of saying that we will not be spending a lot of time on our appearances and will be hiking outdoors), Steve (me) will hold all the cell phones and only take messages, no sex, no smoking, and no drinking. The point underlying Siph-esihle's humorous performance is that this is a serious event and that the group does not want any distractions.

The retreat is held on October 11 and 12, 2008. A facilitator holds a brief orientation and talks about respect for the wilderness and "camp rules." The facilitator (Philani's friend) introduces choir members to a four-part process for the retreat: experience, reflection, generalization, and application. Then we go to a grassy area nearby, where we sit in a circle and do some ice-breaker and team-building activities in which successful completion of a task depends on group cooperation. One of the tasks splits us into two teams and requires each team to stand with their feet on two boards with ropes attached. We have to walk across the grass, which means that all of us have to raise our left foot at the same time and then our right foot at the same time, pulling on the attached ropes with our hands to raise and move the boards as we walk. We have a lot of fun, teasing and joking as we work to coordinate our actions, and we start racing to see who can finish first.

Afterward, our facilitator asks us why we thought of it as a competition? Group members respond by talking about how they get so caught up in things that they lose sight of why they are doing it in the first place. This is also a commentary on group members' feeling about the current state of the choir, and a good start to the retreat.

Next, we pick up our lunches and go on a long hike. When we return to the dormitory to clean up, Philani starts to joke about how he is about to die. He tells group members what he wants them to wear at his funeral, playfully saying things like, "the women should wear brown bras." Philani is joking like this because he is just starting to take antiretroviral medications (ARVs). Group members begin teasing Philani about this fact, saying he will go "straight to the third regimen." This teasing relies on detailed, intimate knowledge of ARV treatment, in which there are first, second, and third "lines" or "regimens" of medications. The general sense is that one progresses to the second and then third regimens when the previous regimen is not working. The choir members' teasing, then, suggests that Philani's life will be cut short because the virus will not respond to available medications. A little later, Amahle tells me that I need to keep my phone handy because no one else is allowed to have theirs, and people need to take their pills at six o'clock, seven o'clock, and nine o'clock. When we eat dinner, I notice that Zethu is eating by herself inside and not really responding to me. Philani explains that she is feeling high and out of sorts after taking a particular ARV pill called Stochrin.

After we cook and eat dinner, Philani pulls me aside. He explains that they are going to have a group meeting where each person talks about his or her commitments. He tells me that I am welcome to join them, but that they will be speaking almost entirely in isiZulu (and not translating for me or switching into English to orient toward me as an audience) so that people can express themselves fully. I decide not to attend the event, thinking that the most ethical thing I can do is to not prioritize my research at the expense of research participants—that is, to give the choir space and privacy to be able to work things out with one another.

The next morning, after breakfast, I go with the group to their morning meeting. Today, they seem to be all business, with Fanele in charge delegating authority. She asks me to set up a Myspace page for the group, to create an email account for the choir, and to teach Amahle and a few other choir members how to use the Internet and set up email accounts for them. Siphesihle is going to be in charge of musical programming—Fanele implores him to be serious about it. Bongiwe will be the finance person since Philani is now living in Pietermaritzburg. They will have a home office in Fanele's apartment. Finally, Sthembile will work to incorporate her sports activism with kids into choir activities. The general idea is to reconstitute the group as a loose organization for support and activism with less of an emphasis on musical performance. Everyone agrees to meet again at the end of November to see how things are going, and then to meet in May 2009 to evaluate the new direction of the group and decide whether or not to continue on this path.

As mentioned earlier in the book, by the time I returned to South Africa in 2013 the choir had stopped operating as a performance and activist group, though many group members continued to stay in close contact and to be supportive of one another. In one sense, the choir had perhaps come to its inevitable conclusion. It had provided a space for support and medical care at a time when that was not generally available; it had yielded a structure for engagement with global health and international aid, soliciting donations and interest that were significantly tied to a number of medical studies and an infusion of resources into South African responses to the epidemic; and it had guided many group members in their treatment to the point where they were taking ARVs and had what they called "full-blown AIDS." By 2008, choir members could collect their ARVs and receive treatment from government-provided medical care, and a number of them had solidified their engagement with global health and worked in (mostly low-paying) positions as HIV counselors.

Still, it was clear that group members were not satisfied with these arrangements. In my view, the natural next step for the choir would have been to continue on in the manner determined at the retreat. A number of group members had crafted innovative, culturally sensitive ideas about future HIV support and activism in their home communities, and the choir might have provided the necessary organization to implement these ideas. Unfortunately, global health groups tended to devalue culturally oriented ideas for prevention (such as those suggested by choir members) in comparison with direct biomedical interventions. Furthermore, choir members lacked the bureaucratic skills needed to function as an independent nonprofit entity. Lastly, doctors and global health professionals tended to restrict choir members and others living with HIV to the patient and/or "cultural expert" roles, and these were roles that were positioned hierarchically below the doctor/researcher roles in global health models. These factors conspired to limit the choir's ability to grow and change, ultimately leading to the disbanding of the group.

The Thembeka choir had initially formed through a love of singing and music, a common Zulu linguacultural heritage, an engagement with influential global health networks in a context of limited access to health care, and HIV-positive diagnoses amid pervasive stigma. This biosocial group developed a shared verbal repertoire and shared language ideologies that cohered around medical discourses about HIV/AIDS. In other words, the choir became a bio-speech community. Group members transposed biomedical understandings of illness, treatment, and activism into rehearsal, performance, and nonbiomedical health-seeking activities. To a limited extent, they were also able to transpose these understandings into home community social events. Here, the term "transposition" (as a special case of translanguaging) theorizes how language and health were intertwined in complex ways that were simultaneously communicative and experiential; and the addition of the prefix "bio" to yield the bio-speech community concept applies theorizations of biopower to studies of language in medical contexts (see also Briggs 2011 on biocommunicability). Biomedicine entails the unparalleled ability to intervene in physiological processes. This ability sets biomedicine apart from other discourses and ideologies. In recognition of this distinction, I have coined the terms "transposition" and "bio-speech community." This book contributes these concepts to a growing body of new scholarship at the intersection of linguistic, medical, and psychological anthropology (see Briggs and Faudree 2016; Ochs 2012).

Transposition of HIV was relevant in the context of global health interventions and HIV stigma. The perceived power of biomedical explanatory models of the virus, the uneven global circulation of money and medication associated with global health interventions, the unavailability of HIV treatment for many South Africans in the late 1990s, and the intense stigmatization of HIV in home communities were all factors that shaped the choir's shared verbal repertoire and language ideologies. This verbal repertoire included ways of joking about and singing about HIV, and these language ideologies not only privileged biomedical discourses about HIV but also valued HIV disclosure as an individual responsibility. Research participants were paradoxically connected to many global health groups while they were marginalized from them—that is, marginalization was linked to the seeking out of connections with multiple groups. The choir's ways of speaking about HIV and their ideologies about those ways of speaking were part and parcel of their positioning as a bio-speech community at the margins of global health groups and home communities.

A BIO-SPEECH COMMUNITY AT THE MARGINS

Conventional speech communities are said to cohere through frequent inter-action, shared norms of language use or language ideologies, and a shared verbal repertoire. As a bio-speech community, in particular, the Thembeka choir's shared ideologies and repertoire orbited around the gravitational well of biomedicine. That is, their language ideologies and verbal repertoire were shaped by the power of biomedicine to diagnose, treat, provide resources for, and institutionalize HIV. The choir was a not simply a bio-speech commu-nity, though. It was a bio-speech community that was specifically situated at the margins of global health. This positioning made relevant the transposi-tion of HIV, a key practice that crosscut the verbal repertoire of the choir community. This practice was itself shaped by language ideologies rooted in the power of biomedical discourses.

This book has analyzed the role of such biopower in the Thembeka choir's creation and maintenance of language ideologies that (1) privileged biomed-ical discourses and cultural models of HIV—a privileging that was central to the process of HIV transposition—and (2) valued practices of HIV dis-closure associated with global health moral/ethical discourses. These ideol-ogies were relevant in the context of pervasive HIV stigmatization. Stigma included ways of talking about HIV that were particularly nonbiomedical. In South Africa, these ways of talking about HIV marked the virus as foreign and negatively evaluated that foreignness. The choir's ideological privileging of biomedical discourses and global health morality/ethics cannot be fully understood without recognizing these stances as oppositional to such a cul-tural context of othering.

The ideological privileging of biomedical discourses and models of HIV were linked to, but not synonymous with, the economic and curative power of those discourses and models. Having a clear, detailed understanding of the biomedical model of HIV was incredibly useful to choir members in their pluralistic health-seeking behaviors. This understanding helped them to avoid negative impacts of mixing treatment methods. Their expertise also enabled them to engage with global health experts, perform together as an HIV-positive choir, and, in some cases, be hired as HIV counselors. However, group members' ideological commitment to biomedical discourses exceeded these stances and activities when they joked with one another about ARVs, TB, HIV, and other things associated with biomedical understandings of the virus. In rehearsals and other social settings, this ideological commitment was central to the creation and maintenance of a distinct speech community. While not discussed in detail in this book, it is worth noting that there were limits to this commitment imposed by stigma in group members' home communities. This was because a verbal display of knowledge about biomedical understandings of HIV could be construed as a close association with biomedical treatment and thus interpreted as disclosure that one was HIV positive.

The valuing of a moral/ethical discourse of HIV disclosure—a discourse focused on individual rights and responsibilities that was associated with global health—was integral to the maintenance of the Thembeka choir speech community. As with to biomedical understandings of HIV, the discourse of individual disclosure as a responsibility was highly valued in global health settings. While global health professionals' perspectives on biomedicine and disclosure largely aligned with those of the choir, these professionals also acted as gatekeepers who limited the ways that choir members engaged with the world of global health. Often, it seemed that global health professionals did so without a clear recognition of their authority. Rather, their influence remained implicit. Choir members received material and economic benefits that were directly tied to their willingness to disclose their HIV-positive status to researchers, international aid workers, and global health professionals. Transposition of this model of HIV disclosure into home community settings was difficult in part because of the existence of a competing Zulu moral/ethical discourse of social duties and respect. Nonetheless, choir members and others living with HIV oriented toward these powerful audiences—listeners whose implicit positive assessments could result in access to resources that were associated with the uneven global circulation of global health.

The choir's ideological privileging of biomedical discourses (including discourses about disclosure) was enacted in and reproduced through a shared verbal repertoire. That verbal repertoire was centered around the set of linguistic practices for utilizing biomedical discourses across social contexts that I have theorized as HIV transposition. I suggest a definition of transposition as a special case of translanguaging (García 2009) that invokes a configuration of medical pluralism (Baer 2011). In the case of HIV transposition among choir members, biomedical understandings of HIV—and biomedical terminology—were valued and reproduced across linguistic contexts and social activities. Analogous to the ways that the feel of a musical tune may change subtly as it is transposed into different tonal centers, the significance of biomedical discourse shifted subtly as choir members utilized that discourse in choir rehearsals, everyday encounters, social events, and performances.

Joking and singing about HIV were two genres in the choir's shared verbal repertoire in which transposition played a central role. In joking encounters with one another, group members deftly played with biomedical understandings of terms that were linked to HIV, such as tuberculosis, antiretroviral medication, disclosure, and even hegemonic gender norms. As speakers collaboratively crafted this humor, they implicitly demonstrated their knowledge of biomedical models, displayed their willingness to face stigmatization, and reflected on the role of the virus in their lives. Here, confrontations with stigma may have been lessened by both the fact that HIV itself remained implicit and the fact that the joking was collaborative—and thus responsibility for the confrontation was distributed across participants. Similarly, singing about HIV was reflexive as well as deeply embodied and collaborative. The synchronization of bodies and voices in tandem with the lyrical content of the songs being sung yielded a powerful physiological alternative to the experiences of stigmatization and illness. The analysis presented in this book suggests that these features of joking and singing about HIV, in conjunction with the intermediate mode of embodied reflexivity that the genres entailed, were central to the ability of the choir to cohere as a bio-speech community amid stigma.

"If You're Negative, Stay Negative; If You're Positive, Think Positive"

In addition to the theoretical contributions of the terms "transposition" and "bio-speech community," this book has also engaged with the Thembeka choir's orientation toward HIV activism, through such goals as providing a human face of the epidemic, spreading awareness about HIV, and showing others that people with HIV are like anyone else and might not exhibit obvi-ous signs of illness or infection. A key aspect of the choir's agenda was to be positive, not just for their own benefit but as a form of activism. This atti-tude was entextualized in choir song lyrics that emphasized, "if you're nega-tive, stay negative; if you're positive, think positive" (if you're HIV negative, stay HIV negative; if you're HIV positive, think positive). One goal of this book has been to capture this stance. Choir members wanted to demonstrate to others that the virus did not need to be a death sentence, that it could be conceptualized as a chronic illness rather than a terminal illness. In my inter-view with her in 2008, Zethu articulated her perspective on this by explain-ing, "God knows what I still have to do in life. And since he gave me [my son], I still have—*ngisafuna uphila* ((I still want to live)) more and more—and see him growing, you know?" In 2018, Zethu's son turned 18. On her Facebook page, she announced this and wrote that she was "feeling positive."

ACKNOWLEDGMENTS

Most special thanks to my parents, who are humanists and scholars, without whom none of this would have been possible; and to Elizabeth Falconi, my partner in life and scholarship, an anthropologist who has read, reread, and talked through almost every idea that appears in this book. Elizabeth also spent two months with me in South Africa in 2008 and contributed immensely to the research process. Thanks also to my brother and sister, Kevin and Alison Black, and to Joe and Betsy Falconi, for their support.

I would like to acknowledge: my transcription assistant, research assistant, and friend, known in my writing as Amahle Ngubane, without whose patience, knowledge, and dialogue this research would have been sorely lacking—*ngiyabonga* (I give praise) to her and her wonderful family; Thembeka choir members for their understanding, friendship, dialogue, and teaching; Talent Mbeje for her tireless work as a transcription assistant; my isiZulu teachers Mary Gordon, Baba Ntshangase, and Zilungile Sosibo for their guidance and patience; and Deva Govindsamy at the U.S. Embassy office in Durban for his guidance as I settled in to the Durban area and made professional contacts.

A very special thanks to Alessandro Duranti, not only for providing unparalleled academic and professional guidance but also for having a sense of humor and some great jazz jam sessions. Thanks to Linda Garro, David Gere, Marjorie Goodwin, Paul Kroskrity, and Elinor Ochs and for their incisive comments and encouragement as advisors while I was at UCLA. Thanks to Robin Conley and Cre Engelke for always making time to read drafts of my work and engage in scholarly dialogue related to my work. Also, thanks to Keith Murphy, Jason Throop, and Suzanne Wertheim for their comments and mentorship. Thanks to the UCLA Discourse Laboratory for listening to and commenting on countless presentations of my work that informed this writing, and to a number of friends and colleagues within and outside that group in particular, including but not limited to Mara Buchbinder, Anna Corwin, Michael Fiorentino, Inmaculada García-Sánchez, Heather Loyd, Lauren Mason Carris, Sonya Pritzker, and Merav Shohet. Thanks to Sam Torrisi for being so Sam, and Daniel Gomez for being very Daniel. I also would like to especially acknowledge the late Brian Ellis, whose friendship and conversations while running on the beaches of Venice and in the Santa Monica Mountains and while hiking and camping through the Sierra Nevada mountains were priceless.

Thank you to a number of colleagues who supported and encouraged me at a time when I was employed in contingent labor positions and as I was working to establish myself as a junior scholar, including Laura Ahearn, Charles Briggs, Paja Faudree, Inmaculada García-Sánchez, Dorothy Hodgson, Bambi Scheiffelin, and Kathryn Woolard. Special thanks to Laura Ahearn (in her role as editor of an Oxford University Press series) whose insight and commentary on a previous draft shaped the current form of the book. Thank you to the many colleagues and mentors who presented on academic panels with me and served as discussants on these panels, inspiring new lines of thought, including co-organizers Anna Corwin, Nathaniel Dumas, and James Wilce. Thanks to Bambi Schieffelin and members of the New York Linguistic Anthropology Working Group and to participants at the Emory African Studies Institute's conference, "Twenty Years Later: South Africa and the Post-Apartheid Condition" for comments on some of this work. Thank you to Lynette Arnold, Netta Avineri, and Xochiquetzal Marsilli-Vargas for commenting on drafts of individual chapters. Finally, thank you to editor Kimberly Guinta at Rutgers University Press and to the anonymous reviewers who provided essential guidance and critique at numerous points throughout the writing process.

This research was made possible by a Doctoral Dissertation Improvement Grant from the National Science Foundation. Some pilot fieldwork was conducted while I was participating in a Zulu Group Project Abroad funded by Fulbright-Hays, organized by the University of Pennsylvania and the University of KwaZulu-Natal. Initial Zulu language learning was funded by a Title VI Foreign Language Area Studies fellowship to attend the Summer Cooperative African Languages Institute at Ohio University administered by the James S. Coleman African Studies Center at the University of California, Los Angeles. Additional funding was provided by the University of California, Los Angeles, Department of Anthropology, and the Georgia State University Department of Anthropology.

NOTES

CHAPTER 1   INTRODUCTION

1. All individuals and organizations that are part of my research are referred to with pseudonyms. This is common anthropological practice in situations where the anonymity of research participants is at issue and is in accordance with institutional review board documents and my agreement with research participants.

2. In this book, I follow South African conventions, using "Zulu" (more appropriately amaZulu) to refer to the ethnic group, and "isiZulu" to refer to the language. The word stem—"Zulu" means above or heavens. In this case, the noun class prefix "isi-" indicates a language (the language of heaven) while the noun class "ama-" indicates a people (the people of heaven).

3. While the term "semiotic transduction" has become popular in linguistic anthropology over the past several years, I tend to avoid the term because I think it can too easily be confused with the primary/ordinary meaning of "transduction," which specifically refers to a conversion from a patterning in the variation of physical quantity to an electrical signal (for more on transduction and its study in an anthropology of sound, see Helmreich 2007).

CHAPTER 2   CONDUCTING ETHNOGRAPHIC FIELDWORK AMID GLOBALIZED INEQUITIES AND STIGMA

1. Afrikaans is a language variety related to sixteenth-century Dutch. It developed among Dutch settlers (sometimes called Boers—"farmers") in interaction with southern African languages and is the result of linguistic convergence and drift away from Dutch. Many Dutch speakers say they can understand much of Afrikaans.

2. Some anthropologists might consider it proper to live with or closer to research participants. In my case, practical concerns prevented me from doing so. No research participants had extra room for me in their homes. Some participants' two-bedroom township homes had as many as six or seven family members already living there. Others lived in even smaller homes or shacks. Another option might have been to find a room to rent somewhere else in the township, but this would have opened up the possibility of my inadvertent disclosure of participants' HIV statuses to my landlords.

CHAPTER 3   THE EMBODIED REFLEXIVITY OF A BIO-SPEECH COMMUNITY

1. From the supertonic to the tonic.

2. Figures 3.6 and 3.7 are an illustrated musical, linguistic, and bodily transcript of these actions. Readers not literate in Euro-classical music notation can get a sense of the temporal unfolding of the excerpt by following the lyrical transcription toward the bottom of the figure and by noting the time elapsed (rounded to the nearest tenth of a second) indicated in parentheses above the music notation but below the description of bodily and gestural actions. Traced outlines of bodies in white indicate movement on beat one, and in gray indicate beat two of the four-beat cycle.

3. See "Transcription Conventions, Orthography, and Morpheme Labels" in the front matter.

CHAPTER 4   THE POWER OF GLOBAL HEALTH AUDIENCES

1. The cultural ideals that shape how people treat children and illness is a topic in and of itself, one that my research did not address. For more on this subject, see Clemente 2015.

2. This indicates that I am unable to hear the word Bongiwe used here.

CHAPTER 5   HIV TRANSPOSITION AMID THE MULTIPLE EXPLANATORY MODELS OF SCIENCE, FAITH, AND TRADITION

1. It seems possible that this understanding of not mixing ARVs with other medicines was communicated to the support group from which the choir developed, perhaps by the doctor who co-ran (with choir member Fanele) the TB Leaders HIV treatment organization in which *izinyanga* (traditional healers) underwent a certification training program. Certainly, this understanding seems to have developed within the group and been shared widely.

CHAPTER 6   THE LINGUISTIC ANTHROPOLOGY OF STIGMA

1. The word "Other" is typically capitalized to indicate that it is a distinction between social categories of persons. In phenomenology the term typically refers to any other person or entity perceived as a thinking, perceiving subject. In some research, though, "othering" has been used to talk about how people distance themselves through processes of stigmatization (e.g., Jenkins and Carpenter-Song 2008).

2. In this transcription tradition, punctuation is used to try to represent the actual intonational contours of a recorded conversation rather than the conventions of written English. Periods indicate downward intonation, question marks indicate upward intonation, commas indicate downward-upward intonation, brackets indicate overlap (when

two people speak at the same time), single parentheses indicate a transcriber's best guess at a difficult-to-hear phrase, multiple question marks indicate something that is not possible to hear, and double parentheses indicate commentary by the transcriber.

3. This has also been described in the past as a (pre)palatal click.

4. These transformations are numbered for convenience of reference. The numbers do not indicate any suggestion as to their historical, cognitive, or grammatical ordering.

CHAPTER 7   PERFORMANCE AND THE TRANSPOSITION OF A GLOBAL HEALTH ETHICS OF DISCLOSURE

Epigraph: From "An Interview with Zackie Achmat—AIDS Activism in South Africa: Lessons for Asia?" Interview by the TREAT Asia Report http://www.amfar.org/articles /around-the-world/treatasia/older/an-interview-with-zackie-achmat—aids-activism -in-south-africa—lessons-for-asia-/.

1. Netball is a sport similar to basketball that was developed in England in the late 1800s. The ball is similar to a volleyball, there are no backboards behind the rim of the baskets, and there is no dribbling and no contact with ball-handlers allowed. It is primarily played in former commonwealth countries, especially at schools, and primarily (but not exclusively) played by women.

2. Ululating is a high-pitched yell during which persons move their tongue up and down against the roof of their mouth to produce something that resembles a series of "la" sounds (or "ula" sounds). In some cultural contexts, ululation accompanies sorrow or anger. In South Africa, it was considered traditional for women to ululate in celebration.

3. *Sanibonani* means "I see you all," in isiZulu, while *yebo* means "yes." This is an everyday greeting, which is why I translate both as "hello" here.

REFERENCES

Abu-Lughod, Lila. 1991. "Writing Against Culture." In *Recapturing Anthropology*, edited by R. Fox, 137–162. Santa Fe: School of American Research.

Adams, S. M. 1932. "Hesiod's Pandora." *Classical Review* 46(5):193–196.

Adendorff, Ralph. 2002. "Fanakalo: A Pidgin in South Africa." In *Language in South Africa*, edited by R. Mesthrie, 179–198. New York: Cambridge University Press.

Agha, Asif. 1998. "Stereotypes and Registers of Honorific Language." *Language in Society* 27(2):151–194.

Allan, Keith, and Kate Burridge. 2006. *Forbidden Words: Taboo and the Censoring of Language*. Cambridge: Cambridge University Press.

Appadurai, Arjun. 1996. *Modernity at Large: Cultural Dimensions of Globalization*. Minneapolis: University of Minnesota Press.

Appalraju, Dhalialutchmee, and Elizabeth de Kadt. 2002. "Gender Aspects of Bilingualism: Language Choice Patterns of Zulu-Speaking Rural Youth. *Southern African Linguistics and Applied Language Studies* 20:135–145.

Aquinas, St. Thomas. 2006 [13th century]. *Summa Theologiae*, vol. 33: *Hope*: 2a2ae. 17–22. New York: Cambridge University Press.

Aristotle. 1998 [4th century B.C.E.]. *The Nicomachean Ethics*. Translated by D. Ross. New York: Oxford University Press.

Ashforth, Adam. 1998. "Reflections on Spiritual Insecurity in a Modern African City (Soweto)." *African Studies Review* 41(3):39–67.

———. 2005. *Witchcraft, Violence, and Democracy in South Africa*. Chicago: University Of Chicago Press.

———. 2011. "AIDS, Religious Enthusiasm and Spiritual Insecurity in Africa." *Global Public Health* 6(2):S132–S147.

Augustine. 1998 [5th century]. *Confessions*. Translated by H. Chadwick. New York: Oxford University Press.

Avineri, Netta. 2017. "Contested Stance Practices in Secular Yiddish Metalinguistic Communities: Negotiating Closeness and Distance." *Journal of Jewish Languages* 5(2):174–199.

Avineri, Netta, and Paul Kroskrity. 2014. "On the (Re-)Production and Representation of Endangered Language Communities: Social Boundaries and Temporal Borders." *Language and Communication* 38(September):1–7.

Baer, Hans A. 2011. "Medical Pluralism: An Evolving and Contested Concept in Medical Anthropology." In *A Companion to Medical Anthropology*, edited by M. Singer and P. I. Erickson, 405–424. Malden, MA: Wiley-Blackwell.

Baer, Hans A., Merrill Singer, and Ida Susser. 2003. *Medical Anthropology and the World System: A Critical Perspective*. 2nd ed. Westport, CT: Praeger.

Banda, Felix. 2018. "Translanguaging and English-African Language Mother Tongues as Linguistic Dispensation in Teaching and Learning in a Black Township School in Cape Town." *Current Issues in Language Planning* 19(2):198–217.

Barrett, Rusty. 2014. "The Emergence of the Unmarked: Queer Theory, Language Ideology, and Formal Linguistics." In *Queer Excursions: Retheorizing Binaries in Language, Gender, and Sexuality*, edited by L. Zimman, J. L. Davis, and J. Raclaw, 195–224. Oxford: Oxford University Press.

Barz, Gregory. 2006. *Singing for Life: HIV/ AIDS and Music in Uganda.* New York: Routledge.

Barz, Gregory, and Judah M. Cohen, eds. 2011. *The Culture of AIDS in Africa: Hope and Healing through Music and the Arts.* New York: Oxford University Press.

Basso, Keith H. 1979. *Portraits of "the Whiteman": Linguistic Play and Cultural Symbols among the Western Apache.* New York: Cambridge University Press.

———. 1988 "'Stalking with Stories': Names, Places, and Moral Narratives among the Western Apache." In *Text, Play, and Story*, edited by E. M. Bruner, 19–55. Washington, DC: American Ethnological Society.

Bauman, Richard. 1975. "Verbal Art as Performance." *American Anthropologist* 77(2): 290–311.

Bauman, Richard, and Charles L. Briggs. 1990. "Poetics and Performance as Critical Perspectives on Language and Social Life." *Annual Review of Anthropology* 19:59–88.

Becker, Judith. 2004. *Deep Listeners: Music, Emotion, and Trancing.* Bloomington: Indiana University Press.

Bell, Allan. 1984. "Language Style as Audience Design." *Language in Society* 13(2): 145–204.

———. 2011. "Falling in Love Again and Again: Marlene Dietrich and the Iconization of Non-Native English." *Journal of Sociolinguistics* 15(5):627–656.

Bell, Allan, and Andy Gibson, eds. 2011. "Staging Language: An Introduction to the Sociolinguistics of Performance." Special issue, *Journal of Sociolinguistics* 15(5).

Benton, Adia. 2015. *HIV Exceptionalism: Development through Disease in Sierra Leone.* Minneapolis: University of Minnesota Press.

Berger, Harris, and Giovanna Del Negro. 2002. "Bauman's Verbal Art and the Social Organization of Attention: The Role of Reflexivity in the Aesthetics of Performance." *Journal of American Folklore* 115(455):62–91.

Berglund, Axel-Ivar. 1976. *Zulu Thought-Patterns and Symbolism.* Cape Town, South Africa: David Philip.

Besnier, Niko. 2004. "The Social Production of Abjection: Desire and Silencing among Transgender Tongans." *Social Anthropology* 12(3):301–323.

———. 2011. *On the Edge of the Global: Modern Anxieties in a Pacific Island Nation.* Stanford: Stanford University Press.

Biehl, João, and Adriana Petryna, eds. 2013. *When People Come First: Critical Studies in Global Health.* Princeton: Princeton University Press.

Black, Steven P. 2013. "Narrating Fragile Stories About HIV/AIDS in South Africa." *Pragmatics and Society* 4(3):345–368.

———. 2018. "Sexual Stigma: Markedness, Taboo, Containment, and Emergence." In *The Oxford Handbook of Language and Sexuality*, edited by K. Hall and R. Barrett. New York: Oxford University Press. https://doi.org/10.1093/oxfordhb/9780190212926 .013.8.

Blommaert, Jan. 2013. *Ethnography, Superdiversity and Linguistic Landscapes: Chronicles of Complexity*. Buffalo: Multilingual Matters.

Boellstorff, Tom. 2009. "Nuri's Testimony: HIV/AIDS in Indonesia and Bare Knowledge." *American Ethnologist* 36(2):351–363.

Bogen, James. 1987. "Finding an Audience." *IPrA Papers in Pragmatics* 1(2):35–65.

Brada, Betsey Behr. 2011. "'Not Here': Making the Spaces and Subjects of 'Global Health' in Botswana." *Culture, Medicine, and Psychiatry* 35(2):285–312.

———. 2017. "Exemplary or Exceptional? The Production and Dismantling of Global Health in Botswana." In *Global Health and Geographical Imaginaries*, edited by Clare Herrick and David Reubi, 40–53. New York: Routledge.

Brenneis, Donald. 1988. "Telling Troubles: Narrative, Conflict and Experience." *Anthropological Linguistics* 30(3/4):279–291.

Briggs, Charles L. 1993. "Personal Sentiments and Polyphonic Voices in Warao Women's Ritual Wailing: Music and Poetics in Critical and Collective Discourse." *American Anthropologist* 95(4):929–957.

———. 2011. "Biocommunicability." In *A Companion to Medical Anthropology*, edited by M. Singer and P. I. Erickson, 459–476. Malden: Wiley-Blackwell.

Briggs, Charles L., and Paja Faudree. 2016. "Communicating Bodies: New Juxtapositions of Linguistic and Medical Anthropology." *Anthropology News* 57:e7–e8.

Briggs, Charles L., and Daniel C. Hallin. 2016. *Making Health Public: How News Coverage is Remaking Media, Medicine, and Contemporary Life*. New York: Routledge.

Briggs, Charles L., and Clara Mantini-Briggs. 2016. *Tell Me Why My Children Died: Rabies, Indigenous Knowledge, and Communicative Justice*. Durham, NC: Duke University.

Brookes, Heather J. 2011. "Amagama Amathathu 'The Three Letters': The Emergence of a Quotable Gesture (Emblem)." *Gesture* 11(2):194–218.

Buchbinder, Mara. 2011. "Personhood Diagnostics: Personal Attributes and Clinical Explanations of Pain." *Medical Anthropology Quarterly* 25(4):457–478.

Bucholtz, Mary. 1999. "'Why Be Normal?' Language and Identity Practices in a Community of Nerd Girls." *Language in Society* 28(2):208–223.

———. 2011. *White Kids: Language, Race, and Styles of Youth Identity*. New York: Cambridge University Press.

———. 2016. "On Being Called Out of One's Name: Indexical Bleaching as a Technique of Deracialization." In *Raciolinguistics: How Language Shapes Our Ideas about Race*, edited by H. S. Alim, J. R. Rickford, and A. F. Ball, 273–289. New York: Oxford University Press.

Bucholtz, Mary, and Kira Hall. 2004. "Language and Identity." In *A Companion to Linguistic Anthropology*, edited by A. Duranti, 369–394. Malden, MA: Blackwell.

———. 2005. "Identity and Interaction: A Sociocultural Linguistic Approach." *Discourse Studies* 7(4–5):585–614.

Bulled, Nicola L. 2015. *Prescribing HIV Prevention: Bringing Culture into Global Health Communication*. Walnut Creek, CA: Left Coast Press.

Cabrita, Joel. 2014. *Text and Authority in the South African Nazaretha Church*. New York: Cambridge University Press.

Capps, Lisa, and Elinor Ochs. 1995. *Constructing Panic: The Discourse of Agoraphobia*. Cambridge, MA: Harvard University Press.

Carr, E. Summerson. 2009. "Anticipating and Inhabiting Institutional Identities." *American Ethnologist* 36(2):317–336.

———. 2010. *Scripting Addiction: The Politics of Therapeutic Talk and American Sobriety*. Princeton: Princeton University Press.

Ciekawy, Diane, and Peter Geschiere, eds. 1998. "Containing Witchcraft: Conflicting Scenarios in Postcolonial Africa." Special issue, *African Studies Review* 41(3).

Clark, Jude. 2006. "The Role of Language and Gender in the Naming and Framing of HIV/AIDS in the South African Context." *Southern African Linguistics and Applied Language Studies* 24(4):461–471.

Clayton, Martin, Rebecca Sager, and Udo Will. 2004. In Time with the Music: The Concept of Entrainment and Its Significance for Ethnomusicology. *ESEM CounterPoint* 1:1–45.

Clemente, Ignasi. 2015. *Uncertain Futures: Communication and Culture in Childhood Cancer Treatment*. Malden, MA: Wiley-Blackwell.

Clemente Pesudo, Ignasi. 2005. "Negotiating the Limits of Uncertainty and Non-Disclosure: Communication and Culture in the Management of Pediatric Cancer Treatment in Barcelona." PhD diss., University of California, Los Angeles.

———. 2007. "Clinicians' Routine Use of Non-Disclosure: Prioritizing 'Protection' Over the Information Needs of Adolescents with Cancer." *Canadian Journal of Nursing Research* 39(4):19–34.

Comaroff, Jean. 2007. "Beyond Bare Life: AIDS, (Bio)Politics, and the Neoliberal Order." *Public Culture* 19(1):197–219.

Comaroff, Jean, and John Comaroff. 1991. *Of Revelation and Revolution: Christianity, Colonialism, and Consciousness in South Africa*. Vol. 1. Chicago: University of Chicago Press.

Comaroff, John, and Jean Comaroff. 1992. *Ethnography and the Historical Imagination*. Boulder: Westview Press.

———. 2004. "Criminal Justice, Cultural Justice: The Limits of Liberalism and the Pragmatics of Difference in the New South Africa." *American Ethnologist* 31(2): 188–204.

———. 2009. *Ethnicity, Inc.* Chicago: University of Chicago Press.

Connell, R. W., and James W. Messerschmidt. 2005. "Hegemonic Masculinity: Rethinking the Concept." *Gender and Society* 19(6):829–859.

Coplan, David. 2007. *In Township Tonight! Three Centuries of South African Black City Music and Theatre*. Auckland Park, South Africa: Jacana Media.

Corrigan, Patrick W., Amy C. Watson, Gabriela Gracia, Natalie Slopen, Kenneth Rasinski, and Laura Hall. 2005. "Newspaper Stories as Measures of Structural Stigma." *Psychiatric Services* 56(5):551–556.

Crapanzano, Vincent. 2003. "Reflections on Hope as a Category of Social and Psychological Analysis." *Cultural Anthropology* 18(1):3–32.

Crimp, Douglas. 1987. "AIDS: Cultural Analysis/Cultural Activism." *October* 43(Winter):3–16.

Csordas, Thomas J. 1994. "Introduction: The Body as Representation and Being-in-the-World." In *Embodiment and Experience*, edited by T. J. Csordas, 1–24. New York: Cambridge University Press.

Davis, Mark, and Lenore Manderson. 2014. "Contours of Truth." In *Disclosure in Health and Illness*, edited by M. Davis and L. Manderson, 153–166. New York: Routledge.

De Klerk, Vivian, and Irene Lagonikos. 2004. "First-Name Changes in South Africa: The Swing of the Pendulum." *International Journal of the Sociology of Language* 170:59–80.

Demuth, Katherine. 2000. "Bantu Noun Class Systems: Loanword and Acquisition Evidence of Semantic Productivity." In *Systems of Nominal Classification*, edited by G. Senft, 270–292. New York: Cambridge University Press.

Dent, G. R., and C. L. S. Nyembezi. 1969. *Scholar's Zulu Dictionary*. Pietermaritzburg, South Africa: Suter & Shooter.

Desjarlais, Robert. R. 1992. *Body and Emotion: The Aesthetics of Illness and Healing in the Nepal Himalayas*. Philadelphia: University of Pennsylvania Press.

Desjarlais, Robert. R., and C. Jason Throop. 2011. "Phenomenological Approaches in Anthropology." *Annual Review of Anthropology* 40:87–102.

Doke, Clement M. 1930 [1927]. *Textbook of Zulu Grammar*. Cape Town, South Africa: Longman Southern Africa.

Douglas, Mary. 1966. *Purity and Danger: An Analysis of Pollution and Taboo*. London: Routledge & Kegan Paul.

Du Bois, W.E.B. 2008 [1903]. *The Souls of Black Folk*. Rockville, MD: ARC Manor.

Duggan, Lisa. 2002. "The New Homonormativity: The Sexual Politics of Neoliberalism." In *Materializing Democracy: Toward a Revitalized Cultural Politics*, edited by R. Castronovo and D. D. Nelson, 175–194. Durham, NC: Duke University Press.

Duranti, Alessandro. 1986. "The Audience as Co-Author." *Text* 6(3):239–247.

———. 1994. *From Grammar to Politics: Linguistic Anthropology in a Western Samoan Village*. Los Angeles: University of California Press.

———. 2006. "Transcripts, Like Shadows on a Wall." *Mind, Culture, and Activity* 13(4):301–310.

Duranti, Alessandro, and Donald Brenneis, eds. 1986. "The Audience As Co-Author." Special issue, *Text* 6(3).

Eckert, Penelope, and Sally McConnell-Ginet. 1998. "Communities of Practice: Where Language, Gender, and Power All Life." In *Language and Gender: A Reader*, edited by J. Coates, 484–494. Oxford: Blackwell.

Elphick, Richard, and Rodney Davenport, eds. 1997. *Christianity in South Africa: A Political, Social, and Cultural History*. Los Angeles: University of California Press.

Erlmann, Veit. 1999. *Music, Modernity and the Global Imagination*. Oxford: Oxford University Press.

Evans-Pritchard, E. E. 1937. *Witchcraft, Oracles and Magic among the Azande*. Oxford: Clarendon Press.

Falconi, Elizabeth. 2013. "Storytelling, Language Shift, and Revitalization in a Transborder Community: 'Tell It in Zapotec!'" *American Anthropologist* 115(4):622–636.

Fassin, Didier. 2007. *When Bodies Remember: Experiences and Politics of AIDS in South Africa*. Los Angeles: University of California Press.

———. 2009. "Another Politics of Life Is Possible." *Theory, Culture and Society* 26(5):44–60.

———. 2011. *Humanitarian Reason: A Moral History of the Present*. Los Angeles: University of California Press.

———. 2012. "That Obscure Object of Global Health." In *Medical Anthropology at the Intersections*, edited by M. C. Inhorn and E. A. Wentzell, 95–115. Durham, NC: Duke University Press.

Fassin, Didier, and Helen Schneider. 2003. "The Politics of AIDS in South Africa: Beyond the Controversies." *BMJ: British Medical Journal* 326(7387):495–497.

Feld, Steven. 1988. "Notes on World Beat." *Public Culture* 1(1):31–37.

Feld, Steven, and Aaron A. Fox. 1994. "Music and Language." *Annual Review of Anthropology* 23:25–53.

Feld, Steven, Aaron A. Fox, Thomas Porcello, and David Samuels. 2004. "Vocal Anthropology: From the Music of Language to the Language of Song." In *A Companion to Linguistic Anthropology*, edited by A. Duranti, 321–346. Malden, MA: Blackwell.

Finlayson, Rosalie. 2002. "Women's Language of Respect: Isihlonipho Sabafazi." In *Language in South Africa*, edited by R. Mesthrie, 279–296. New York: Cambridge University Press.

Fleming, Luke, and Michael Lempert, eds. 2011. "The Unmentionable: Verbal Taboo and the Moral Life of Language." Special issue, *Anthropological Quarterly* 84(1).

Foucault, Michel. 1965 [1961]. *The Birth of the Clinic: An Archaeology of Medical Perception*. New York: Vintage.

———. 1978. *The History of Sexuality*. New York: Pantheon Books.

———. 1979. *Discipline and Punish: The Birth of the Prison*. New York: Vintage Books.

———. 1986. *The Care of the Self*. The History of Sexuality, vol. 3. Translated by R. Hurley. New York: Random House.

———. 1993. "On the Genealogy of Ethics: An Overview of Work in Progress." In *The Essential Foucault: Selections from the Essential Works of Foucault 1954–1984*, edited by P. Rabinow and N. Rose, 102–125. New York: The New Press.

Friedner, Michele. 2010. "Biopower, Biosociality, and Community Formation: How Biopower Is Constitutive of the Deaf Community." *Sign Language Studies* 10(3):336–347.

García, Angela. 2014. "The Promise: On the Morality of the Marginal and the Illicit." *Ethos* 42(1):51–64.

García, Ofelia. 2009. "Education, Multilingualism and Translanguaging in the 21st Century." In *Multilingual Education for Social Justice: Globalising the Local*, edited by Ajit Mohanty, Minati Panda, Robert Phillipson, and Tove Skutnabb-Kangas, 128–145. New Delhi: Orient Blackswan.

Garro, Linda C. 2000. "Cultural Meaning, Explanations of Illness, and the Development of Comparative Frameworks." *Ethnology* 39(4):305–334.

———. 2002. "Hallowell's Challenge: Explanations of Illness and Cross-Cultural Research." *Anthropological Theory* 2(1):77–97.

———. 2011. "Enacting Ethos, Enacting Health: Realizing Health in the Everyday Life of a California Family of Mexican Descent." *Ethos* 39(3):300–330.

Gaudio, Rudolf. 2009. *Allah Made Us: Sexual Outlaws in an Islamic African City*. Malden, MA: Wiley-Blackwell.

Gilroy, Paul. 1993. *The Black Atlantic: Modernity and Double Consciousness*. Cambridge, MA: Harvard University Press.

Goffman, Erving. 1963. *Stigma: Notes on the Management of Spoiled Identity*. Englewood Cliffs, NJ: Prentice-Hall.

———. 1974. *Frame Analysis: An Essay on the Organization of Experience*. Boston: Northeastern University Press.

Good, Byron J. 1994. *Medicine, Rationality, and Experience: An Anthropological Perspective*. Cambridge: Cambridge University Press.

Goodwin, Marjorie. 1990. *He-Said-She-Said: Talk as Social Organization among Black Children*. Bloomington: Indiana University Press.

Goodwin, Marjorie, and Charles Goodwin. 2000. "Emotions within Situated Activity." In *Communication: An Arena of Development*, edited by N. Bidwig, I. C. Uzigiris, and J. V. Wertsch, 33–53. Westport, CT: Greenwood Publishing Group.

Guell, Cornelia. 2011. "Candi(ed) Action: Biosocialities of Turkish Berliners Living with Diabetes." *Medical Anthropology Quarterly* 25(3):377–394.

Gumperz, John. 1972. "The Speech Community." In *Language and Social Context*, edited by P. P. Giglioli, 219–231. Harmondsworth: Penguin.

———. 1982. *Discourse Strategies*. New York: Cambridge University Press.

Guzmán, Jennifer R. 2014. "The Epistemics of Symptom Experience and Symptom Accounts in Mapuche Healing and Pediatric Primary Care in Southern Chile." *Journal of Linguistic Anthropology* 24(3):249–276.

Hall, Kira. 2004. "Language and Marginalized Places." In *Language and Woman's Place: Text and Commentaries*, edited by M. Bucholtz, 171–177. New York: Oxford University Press.

Hall, Kira, and Veronica O'Donovan. 1996. "Shifting Gender Positions among Hindi-Speaking Hijras." In *Rethinking Language and Gender Research: Theory and Practice*, edited by V. Bergvall, J. Bing, and A. Freed, 228–266. New York: Taylor and Francis.

Hankins, Joseph. 2014. *Working Skin: Making Leather, Making a Multicultural Japan*. Los Angeles: University of California Press.

Hanks, William F. 2010. *Converting Words: Maya in the Age of the Cross*. Los Angeles: University of California Press.

Hansen, Thomas Blom. 2012. *Melancholia of Freedom: Social Life in an Indian Township in South Africa*. Princeton: Princeton University Press.

Harvey, T. S. 2013. *Wellness Beyond Words: Maya Compositions of Speech and Silence in Medical Care*. Albuquerque: University of New Mexico Press.

Helmreich, Stefan. 2007. "An Anthropologist Underwater: Immersive Soundscapes, Submarine Cyborgs, and Transductive Ethnography." *American Ethnologist* 34(4):621–641.

Herbert, Robert K. 1990a. "The Relative Markedness of Click Sounds: Evidence from Language Change, Acquisition, and Avoidance." *Anthropological Linguistics* 32(1–2):120–138.

———. 1990b. "The Sociohistory of Clicks in Southern Bantu." *Anthropological Linguistics* 32:295–315.

Hinton, Devon, and Laurence J. Kirmayer. 2017. "The Flexibility Hypothesis of Healing." *Culture, Medicine, and Psychiatry* 41(1):3–34.

Hörbst, Viola, and Trudie Gerrits. 2016. "Transnational Connections of Health Professionals: Medicoscapes and Assisted Reproduction in Ghana and Uganda." *Ethnicity and Health* 21(4):357–374.

Hunter, Mark. 2005. "Cultural Politics and Masculinities: Multiple-Partners in Historical Perspective in KwaZulu-Natal." *Culture, Health & Sexuality* 7(4):389–403.

———. 2007. "The Changing Political Economy of Sex in South Africa: The Significance of Unemployment and Inequalities to the Scale of the AIDS Pandemic." *Social Science & Medicine* 64(2007):689–700.

———. 2010. *Love in the Time of AIDS: Inequality, Gender, and Rights in South Africa.* Bloomington: Indiana University Press.

Inhorn, Marcia C., and Emily A. Wentzell. 2011. "Embodying Emergent Masculinities: Men Engaging with Reproductive and Sexual Health Technologies in the Middle East and Mexico." *American Ethnologist* 38(4):801–815.

Inoue, Miyako. 2003. "The Listening Subject of Japanese Modernity and His Auditory Double: Citing, Sighting, and Siting the Modern Japanese Woman." *Cultural Anthropology* 18(2):156–193.

Irvine, Judith. 1998. "Ideologies of Honorific Language." In *Language Ideologies: Practice and Theory,* edited by B. Schieffelin, K. Woolard, and P. Kroskrity, 51–67. New York: Oxford University Press.

———. 2011. "Leaky Registers and Eight-Hundred-Pound Gorillas." *Anthropological Quarterly* 84(1):15–39.

Irvine, Judith, and Susan Gal. 2000. "Language Ideology and Linguistic Differentiation." In *Regimes of Language: Ideologies, Polities, and Identities,* edited by P. V. Kroskrity, 35–83. Santa Fe, NM: School of American Research.

Jacobs-Huey, Lanita. 2002. "The Natives Are Gazing and Talking Back: Reviewing the Problematics of Positionality, Voice, and Accountability among 'Native' Anthropologists." *American Anthropologist* 104(3):791–804.

Jakobson, Roman. 1959. "Linguistic Aspects of Translation." In *On Translation,* edited by R. A. Brower, 232–239. Cambridge, MA: Harvard University Press.

———. 1960. "Concluding Statement: Linguistics and Poetics." In *Style and Language,* edited by T. A. Sebeok, 350–377. Cambridge, MA: MIT Press.

———. 1990. "The Concept of Mark (with Krystyna Pomorska)." In *On Language,* edited by L. R. Waugh and M. Monville-Burston, 134–140. Cambridge, MA: Harvard University Press.

Jefferson, Gail. 1984. "Notes on Some Orderlinesses of Overlap Onset." In *Discourse Analysis and Natural Rhetorics*, edited by V. D'Urso and P. Leonardi, 11–38. Padua: Cleupe editore.

Jenkins, Janis H., and Elizabeth A. Carpenter-Song. 2008. "Stigma Despite Recovery: Strategies for Living in the Aftermath of Psychosis." *Medical Anthropology Quarterly* 22(4):381–409.

Jolaosho, Omotayo. 2012. "Cross-Circulations and Transnational Solidarity: Historicizing the U.S. Anti-Apartheid Movement through Song." *Safundi: The Journal of South African and American Studies* 13(3–4):317–337.

Jones, Edward E., Amerigo Farina, Albert H. Hastorf, Hazel Markus, Dale T. Miller, and Robert A. Scott. 1984. *Social Stigma: The Psychology of Marked Relationships*. New York: Freeman.

Keane, Webb. 2007. *Christian Moderns: Freedom and Fetish in the Mission Encounter*. Los Angeles: University of California Press.

———. 2011. "Indexing Voice: A Morality Tale." *Journal of Linguistic Anthropology* 21(2):166–178.

King, Brian. 2012. "'We Pray at the Church in the Day and Visit the Sangomas at Night': Health Discourses and Traditional Medicine in Rural South Africa." *Annals of the Association of American Geographers* 102(5):1173–1181.

Kleinman, Arthur. 1978. "Concepts and a Model for the Comparison of Medical Systems as Cultural Systems." *Social Science & Medicine* 12:85–93.

———. 1988. *The Illness Narratives: Suffering, Healing, and the Human Condition*. New York: Basic Books.

———. 2006. *What Really Matters: Living a Moral Life Amidst Uncertainty and Danger*. Oxford: Oxford University Press.

———. 2012. "Medical Anthropology and Mental Health: Five Questions for the Next Fifty Years." In *Medical Anthropology at the Intersections: Histories, Activisms, and Futures*, edited by M. C. Inhorn and E. A. Wentzell, 116–128. Durham, NC: Duke University Press.

Koen, Benjamin D. 2005. "Medical Ethnomusicology in the Pamir Mountains: Music and Prayer in Healing." *Ethnomusicology* 49(2):287–311.

Koen, Benjamin D., Jacqueline Lloyd, Gregory Barz, and Karen Brummel-Smith, eds. 2008. *The Oxford Handbook of Medical Ethnomusicology*. New York: Oxford University Press.

Koopman, Adrian. 2002. *Zulu Names*. Durban, South Africa: University of KwaZulu-Natal Press.

Kuipers, Joel C. 1989. "'Medical Discourse' in Anthropological Context: Views of Language and Power." *Medical Anthropology Quarterly* 3(2):99–123.

Kuper, Adam. 2003. "The Return of the Native." *Current Anthropology* 44:389–402.

Lambek, Michael, ed. 2010. *Ordinary Ethics: Anthropology, Language, and Action*. New York: Fordham University Press.

Langwick, Stacy. 2007. "Devils, Parasites, and Fierce Needles: Healing and the Politics of Translation in Southern Tanzania." *Science, Technology and Human Values* 32(1): 88–117.

Leclerc-Madlala, Suzanne, Leickness C. Simbayi, and Allanise Cloete. 2009. "The Socio-cultural Aspects of HIV/AIDS in South Africa." In *HIV/AIDS in South Africa 25 Years On: Psychosocial Perspectives*, edited by P. Rohleder, L. Swartz, S. Kalichman, and L. C. Simbayi, 13–26. New York: Springer.

Liang, A. C. 1997. "The Creation of Coherence in Coming-Out Stories." In *Queerly Phrased: Language, Gender, and Sexuality*, edited by A. Livia and K. Hall, 287–309. New York: Oxford University Press.

Link, Bruce G., and Jo C. Phelan. 2001. "Conceptualizing Stigma." *Annual Review of Sociology* 27:363–385.

Lønsmann, Dorte, Spencer Hazel, and Hartmut Haberland. 2017. "Introduction to Special Issue on Transience: Emerging Norms of Language Use." *Journal of Linguistic Anthropology* 27(3):264–270.

Lucy, John. 2000. "Systems of Nominal Classification: A Concluding Discussion." In *Systems of Nominal Classification*, edited by G. Senft, 326–341. New York: Cambridge University Press.

Mamdani, Mahmood. 1996. *Citizen and Subject: Contemporary Africa and the Legacy of Late Colonialism*. Princeton: Princeton University Press.

Marsilli-Vargas, Xochitl. 2014. "Listening Genres: The Emergence of Relevance Structures through the Reception of Sound." *Journal of Pragmatics* 69:42–51.

Marsland, Rebecca. 2012. "(Bio)Sociality and HIV in Tanzania." *Medical Anthropology Quarterly* 26(4):470–485.

Mattingly, Cheryl. 1998. *Healing Dramas and Clinical Plots: The Narrative Structure of Experience*. Cambridge: Cambridge University Press.

———. 2010. *The Paradox of Hope: Journeys through a Clinical Borderland*. Berkeley: University of California Press.

Mattingly, Cheryl, and Linda C. Garro, eds. 2000. *Narrative and the Cultural Construction of Illness and Healing*. Los Angeles: University of California Press.

Mbeje, Audrey N. 2005. *Zulu Learner's Reference Grammar*. Madison, WI: National African Language Resource Center Press.

McCormick, Kay. 2002. *Language in Cape Town's District Six*. Oxford: Oxford University Press.

McNeill, Fraser. 2011. *AIDS, Politics, and Music in South Africa*. New York: Cambridge University Press.

Meintjes, Louise. 2003. *Sound of Africa: Making Music Zulu in a South African Studio*. Durham, NC: Duke University Press.

———. 2004. "Shoot the Sergeant, Shatter the Mountain: The Production of Masculinity in Zulu Ngoma Song and Dance in Post-Apartheid South Africa." *Ethnomusicology Forum* 13(2):173–201.

Mesthrie, R. 2002. "South Africa: A Sociolinguistic Overview." In *Language in South Africa*, edited by R. Mesthrie, 11–26. New York: Cambridge University Press.

Milroy, Leslie. 2002. "Social Networks." In *The Handbook of Language Variation and Change*, edited by J. K. Chambers, P. Trudgill, and N. Schilling-Estes, 549–572. Oxford: Blackwell.

Minkowski, Eugene. 1970. *Lived Time: Phenomenological and Psychopathological Studies.* Translated by N. Metzel. Evanston, IL: Northwestern University Press.

Moolman, Benita. 2013. "Rethinking 'Masculinities in Transition' in South Africa Considering the 'Intersectionality' of Race, Class, and Sexuality with Gender." *African Identities* 11(1):93–105.

Morgan, Marcyleina. 2001. "The African American Speech Community: Reality and Sociolinguistics." In *Linguistic Anthropology: A Reader*, edited by A. Duranti, 74–94. Malden, MA: Blackwell.

———. 2004. "Speech Community." In *A Companion to Linguistic Anthropology*, edited by A. Duranti, 3–22. Malden, MA: Blackwell.

Narayan, Kirin. 1993. "How Native is a 'Native' Anthropologist?" *American Anthropologist* 95:671–685.

Ngubane, Harriet. 1977. *Body and Mind in Zulu medicine: An Ethnography of Health and Disease in Nyuswa-Zulu Thought and Practice.* New York: Academic Press.

Nguyen, Vinh-Kim. 2008. "Antiretroviral Globalism, Biopolitics, and Therapeutic Citizenship." In *Global Assemblages: Technology, Politics, and Ethics as Anthropological Problems*, edited by A. Ong and S. J. Collier, 124–144. Oxford: Blackwell.

———. 2010. *The Republic of Therapy: Triage and Sovereignty in West Africa's Time of AIDS.* Durham, NC: Duke University Press.

Niehaus, Isak A. 1998. "The ANC's Dilemma: The Symbolic Politics of Three Witch-Hunts in the South African Lowveld, 1990–1995." *African Studies Review* 41(3):93–118.

———. 2007. "Death Before Dying: Understanding AIDS Stigma in the South African Lowveld." *Journal of Southern African Studies* 33(4):845–860.

Nietzsche, Friedrich. 1966 [1907]. *Beyond Good and Evil.* Translated by W. Kaufmann. New York: Vintage Books.

Nurse, Derek, and Gerard Philippson, eds. 2003. *The Bantu Languages.* New York: Routledge.

Ochs, Elinor. 1979. "Transcription as Theory." In *Developmental pragmatics*, edited by E. Ochs and B. B. Schieffelin, 43–72. New York: Academic Press.

———. 2012. "Experiencing Language." *Anthropological Theory* 12(2):142–160.

Ochs, Elinor, and Lisa Capps. 1997. "Narrative Authenticity." *Journal of Narrative and Life History* 7(1–4):83–89.

Ong, Aihwa, and Stephen J. Collier, eds. 2008. *Global Assemblages: Technology, Politics, and Ethics as Anthropological Problems.* Oxford: Blackwell.

Oppenheimer, Gerald M., and Ronald Bayer. 2007. *Shattered Dreams? An Oral History of the South African AIDS Epidemic.* Oxford: Oxford University Press.

Parkin, David. 2013. "Medical Crises and Therapeutic Talk." *Anthropology and Medicine* 20(2):124–141.

Penkala-Gawecka, Danuta, and Malgorzata Rajtar. 2016. "Introduction to the Special Issue 'Medical Pluralism and Beyond.'" *Anthropology and Medicine* 23(2):129–134.

Pennebaker, James W. 2003. "Telling Stories: The Health Benefits of Disclosure." In *Social and Cultural Lives of Immune Systems*, edited by J. M. Wilce, 19–35. New York: Routledge.

Pfeiffer, James. 2002. "African Independent Churches in Mozambique: Healing the Afflictions of Inequality." *Medical Anthropology Quarterly* 16(2):176–199.

Pigg, Stacy Leigh. 1997. "Authority in Translation: Finding, Knowing, Naming and Training 'Traditional Birth Attendants' in Nepal." In *Childbirth and Authoritative Knowledge: Cross-Cultural Perspectives*, edited by R. Davis-Floyd and C. F. Sargent, 233–262. Berkeley: University of California Press.

———. 2001. "Languages of Sex and AIDS in Nepal: Notes on the Social Production of Commensurability." *Cultural Anthropology* 16(4):481–541.

Piot, Charles. 2001. "Atlantic Aporias: Africa and Gilroy's Black Atlantic." *South Atlantic Quarterly* 100(1):155–170.

Poulos, George, and Sonja E. Bosch. 1997. *Zulu*. Vol. 50. Newcastle: Lincom Europa.

Poulos, George, and Christian T. Msimang. 1998. *A Linguistic Analysis of Zulu*. Cape Town, South Africa: Via Afrika.

Pritzker, Sonya E. 2014. *Living Translation: Language and the Search for Resonance in U.S. Chinese Medicine*. New York: Berghahn books.

Quinn, Naomi. 2005. "Universals of Child Rearing." *Anthropological Theory* 5(4):477–516.

Rabinow, Paul. 1992. "Artificiality and Enlightenment: From Sociobiology to Biosociality." In *In-Corporations*, edited by J. Crary and S. Kwinter, 234–252. New York: Zone.

Rapp, Rayna. 1999. *Testing Women, Testing the Fetus: The Social Impact of Amniocentesis in America*. New York: Routledge.

Reynolds, Jennifer F., and Marjorie Faulstitch Orellana. 2015. "Translanguaging within Enactments of Quotidian Interpreter-Mediated Interactions." *Journal of Linguistic Anthropology* 24(3):315–338.

Ricoeur, Paul. 1984. *Time and Narrative*. Chicago: University of Chicago Press.

Robbins, Joel. 2004. *Becoming Sinners: Christianity and Moral Torment in a Papua New Guinea Society*. Los Angeles: University of California Press.

———. 2007. "Between Reproduction and Freedom: Morality, Value, and Radical Cultural Change." *Ethnos* 72(2):293–314.

———. 2009. "Value, Structure, and the Range of Possibilities: A Response to Zigon." *Ethnos* 74(2):277–285.

———. 2013. "Beyond the Suffering Subject: Toward an Anthropology of the Good." *Journal of the Royal Anthropological Institute* 19(3):447–462.

Robins, Steven. 2006. "From 'Rights' to 'Ritual': AIDS Activism in South Africa." *American Anthropologist* 108(2):312–323.

———. 2008. *From Revolution to Rights in South Africa: Social Movements, NGOs and Popular Politics after Apartheid*. Pietermaritzburg, South Africa: University of KwaZulu-Natal Press.

Rosenfeld, Dana, and Christopher A. Faircloth, eds. 2006. *Medicalized Masculinities*. Philadelphia: Temple University Press.

Rudwick, Stephanie Inge. 2008. "Shifting Norms of Linguistic and Cultural Respect: Hybrid Sociolinguistic Zulu Identities." *Nordic Journal of African Studies* 17(2): 152–174.

Rumsey, Alan. 2010. "Ethics, Language, and Human Sociality." In *Ordinary Ethics: Anthropology, Language, and Action*, edited by M. Lambek, 105–122. New York: Fordham University Press.

Rymes, Betsy. 1996. "Naming as Social Practice: The Case of Little Creeper from Diamond Street." *Language in Society* 25(2):237–260.

Sacks, Harvey, Emanuel Schegloff, and Gail Jefferson. 1974. "A simplest systematics for the organization of turn-taking for conversation." *Language* 50(4):696–735.

Samuels, David. 2004. *Putting a Song On Top of It: Expression and Identity on the San Carlos Apache Reservation*. Tucson: University of Arizona Press.

Scheper-Hughes, Nancy, and Margaret Lock. 1987. "The Mindful Body: A Prolegomenon to Future Work in Medical Anthropology." *Medical Anthropology Quarterly* 1(1):6–41.

Schieffelin, Bambi. 2007. "Found in Translating: Reflexive Language Across Time and Texts." In *Consequences of Contact: Language Ideologies and Social Transformation in Pacific Societies*, edited by M. Makihara and B. Schieffelin, 140–165. Oxford: Oxford University Press.

Schutz, Alfred. 1964. "Making Music Together: A Study in Social Relationship." In *Alfred Schutz, Collected Papers*, edited by A. Broderson, 159–178. Vol. 2. The Hague: Martinus Nijhoff.

Scourgie, Fiona. 2008. *Plural Health Systems*. Durban, South Africa: Centre for HIV/AIDS Networking (HIVAN), University of KwaZulu-Natal.

Seidel, Gill. 1993. "The Competing Discourses of HIV/AIDS in Sub-Saharan Africa: Discourses of Rights and Empowerment vs. Discourses of Control and Exclusion." *Social Science and Medicine* 36(3):175–194.

Selikow, Terry-Ann. 2004. "'We have our own special language.' Language, sexuality and HIV/ AIDS: A case study of youth in an urban township in South Africa." *African Health Sciences* 4(2):102–108.

Sherzer, Joel. 2002. *Speech Play and Verbal Art*. Austin: University of Texas Press.

Shisana, O., T. Rehle, L. C. Simbayi, K. Zuma, S. Jooste, V. Pillay-Van Wyk, N. Mbelle, J. Van Zyi, W. Parker, N. P. Zungu, S. Pezi, and SABBSSM III Implementation Team. 2009. *South African National HIV Prevalence, Incidence, Behavior and Communication Survey, 2008: A Turning Tide among Teenagers?* Pretoria: Human Sciences Research Council.

Shisana, O., T. Rehle, L. C. Simbayi, K. Zuma, S. Jooste, N. Zungu, D. Labadorios, and D. Onoya. 2014. *South African National HIV Prevalence, Incidence, and Behaviour Survey, 2012*. Cape Town: Human Sciences Research Council Press.

Shohet, Merav. 2007. "Narrating anorexia: 'Full' and 'Struggling' Genres of Recovery." *Ethos* 35(3):344–382.

Shuck, Gail. 2004. "Conversational Performance and the Poetic Construction of an Ideology." *Language in Society* 33(2):195–221.

Silverstein, Michael. 1986. "Classifiers, Verb Classifiers, and Verbal Categories." *Berkeley Linguistics Society* 12:497–514.

———. 2003. "Translation, Transduction, Transformation: Skating 'Glossando' on Thin Semiotic Ice." In *Translating Cultures: Perspectives on Translation and Anthropology*, edited by P. G. Rubel and A. Rosman, 75–105. Oxford: Berg.

Slabbert, S., and R. Finlayson. 2002. "Code-Switching in South African Townships." In *Language in South Africa*, edited by R. Mesthrie, 235–257. New York: Cambridge University Press.

Sontag, Susan. 1989. *Illness as Metaphor and AIDS and Its Metaphors*. New York: Picador.

Speer, Susan. 2001. "Reconsidering the Concept of Hegemonic Masculinity: Discursive Psychology, Conversation Analysis and Participants' Orientations." *Feminism and Psychology* 11(1):107–135.

Spitulnik, Debra. 1996. "The Social Circulation of Media Discourse and the Mediation of Communities." *Journal of Linguistic Anthropology* 6(2):161–187.

Squire, Corinne. 2007. *HIV in South Africa: Talking about the Big Thing*. New York: Routledge.

Stadler, Jonathan. 2003. "Rumor, Gossip and Blame: Implications for HIV/ AIDS Prevention in the South African Lowveld." *AIDS Education and Prevention* 15(4): 357–368.

Steiner, Franz. 1956. *Taboo*. Baltimore, MD: Penguin Books.

Stivers, Tanya. 2007. *Prescribing under Pressure: Parent–Physician Conversations and Antibiotics*. New York: Oxford University Press.

Strauss, Claudia, and Naomi Quinn. 1997. *A Cognitive Theory of Cultural Meaning*. Cambridge: Cambridge University Press.

Streeck, Jurgen, Charles Goodwin, and C. LeBaron, eds. 2012. *Embodied Interaction: Language and Body in the Material World*. New York: Cambridge University Press.

Susser, Ida. 2009. *AIDS, Sex, and Culture: Global Politics and Survival in Southern Africa*. Malden, MA: Wiley-Blackwell.

Suzman, Susan M. 1994. "Names as Pointers: Zulu Personal Naming Practices." *Language in Society* 23(2):253–272.

Teppo, Annika. 2011. "'Our Spirit Has No Boundary': White Sangomas and Mediation in Cape Town." *Anthropology and Humanism* 36(2):225–247.

Thompson, Leonard. 2000. *A History of South Africa*. New Haven: Yale University Press.

Throop, C. Jason. 2002. "Experience, Coherence, and Culture: The Significance of Dilthey's 'Descriptive Psychology' for the Anthropology of Consciousness." *Anthropology of Consciousness* 13(1):2–26.

———. 2003. "Articulating Experience." *Anthropological Theory* 3(2):219–241.

Treichler, Paula A. 1987. "AIDS, Homophobia, and Biomedical Discourse: An Epidemic of Signification." *October* 43(Winter):31–70.

———. 1999. "AIDS and HIV Infection in the Third World: A First World Chronicle." In *How to Have Theory in an Epidemic: Cultural Chronicles of AIDS*, 99–126. Durham, NC: Duke University Press.

Trubetzkoy, Nikolai Sergeevich. 1969 [1939]. *Principles of Phonology*. Translated by C. A. M. Baltaxe. Los Angeles: University of California Press.

Turino, Thomas. 1999. "Signs of Imagination, Identity, and Experience: A Peircean Semiotic Theory for Music." *Ethnomusicology* 43(2):221–255.

Turner, Victor. 1987. *The Anthropology of Performance*. Baltimore: Johns Hopkins University Press.

Vilakazi, Absolom. 1962. *Zulu Transformations: A Study of the Dynamics of Social Change*. Pietermaritzburg, South Africa: University of Natal Press.

Webster, Anthony K., and Paul V. Kroskrity. 2013. "Introducing Ethnopoetics: Hymes's Legacy." *Journal of Folklore Research* 50(1–3):1–11.

White, Cassandra. 2008. "Iatrogenic Stigma in Outpatient Treatment for Hansen's Disease (Leprosy) in Brazil." *Health Education Research* 23(1):25–39.

Whyte, Susan Reynolds. 2009. "Health Identities and Subjectivities: The Ethnographic Challenge." *Medical Anthropology Quarterly* 23(1):6–15.

Wickström, Anette. 2014. "'Lungisa'—Weaving Relationships and Social Space to Restore Health in Rural KwaZulu Natal." *Medical Anthropology Quarterly* 28(2):203–220.

Wilce, James M., Jr. 2009a. *Crying Shame: Metaculture, Modernity, and the Exaggerated Death of Lament*. Malden, MA: Wiley-Blackwell.

———. 2009b. "Medical Discourse." *Annual Review of Anthropology* 38:199–215.

———. 2017. "Tradition, Emotion, Healing and the Sacred: Revivalist Lamenting in Finland in Relation to Three Authenticities." In *Spirit and Mind: Mental Health at the Intersection of Religion and Psychiatry*, edited by H. Basu, R. Littlewood, and A. S. Steinforth, 227–252. Berlin: Deutsche Nationalbibliothek.

Williams, Quentin E., and Christopher Stroud. 2014. "Battling the Race: Stylizing Language and Colouredness in a Freestyle Rap Performance." *Journal of Linguistic Anthropology* 24(3):277–293.

Wood, Kate, and Helen Lambert. 2008. "Coded Talk, Scripted Omissions: The Micropolitics of AIDS Talk in an Affected Community in South Africa." *Medical Anthropology Quarterly* 22(3):213–233.

Woolard, Kathryn. 1998. "Simultaneity and Bivalency as Strategies in Bilingualism." *Journal of Linguistic Anthropology* 8(1):3–29.

———. 2004. "Codeswitching." In *A Companion to Linguistic Anthropology*, edited by A. Duranti, 73–94. Malden, MA: Blackwell.

Yang, Lawrence Hsin, et al. 2007. "Culture and Stigma: Adding Moral Experience to Stigma Theory." *Social Science & Medicine* 64(7):1524–1535.

Zentella, Ana Celia. 1997. *Growing Up Bilingual: Puerto Rican Children in New York*. Malden, MA: Blackwell.

Zigon, Jarrett. 2009. "Within a Range of Possibilities: Morality and Ethics in Social Life." *Ethnos* 74(2):251–276.

———. 2011. *"HIV Is God's Blessing": Rehabilitating Morality in Neoliberal Russia*. Berkeley: University of California Press.

Zigon, Jarrett, and C. Jason Throop. 2014. "Moral Experience: Introduction." *Ethos* 42(1):1–15.

INDEX

ABOUT THE AUTHOR

STEVEN P. BLACK is an associate professor of anthropology at Georgia State University, and the lead researcher for the Global Health Discourses Project. He has performed as a professional jazz saxophonist in Australia, South Africa, and the United States.